The Jossey-Bass Health Care Series brings together the most current information and ideas in health care from the leaders in the field. Titles from the Jossey-Bass Health Care Series include these essential health care resources:

After Restructuring: Empowerment Strategies at Work in America's Hospitals,
Thomas G. Rundall, David B. Starkweather, Barbara R. Norrish

Agility in Health Care: Strategies for Mastering Turbulent Markets,
Steven L. Goldman, Carol B. Graham

Board Work: Governing Health Care Organizations,
Dennis D. Pointer, James E. Orlikoff

Clinical Integration: Strategies and Practices for Organized Delivery Systems,
Mary Tonges

Creating the New American Hospital: A Time for Greatness,
V. Clayton Sherman

Health Care Alliances and Conversions: A Handbook for Nonprofit Trustees,
James R. Schwartz, H. Chester Horn, Jr.

Managed Care Contracting: A Practical Guide for Health Care Executives,
William A. Garofalo, Eve T. Horwitz, Thomas M. Reardon

Managing Patient Expectations: The Art of Finding and Keeping Loyal Patients, Susan Keane Baker

Med Inc.: How Consolidation Is Shaping Tomorrow's Healthcare System,
Sandy Lutz, Woodrin Grossman, John Bigalke

Physician Profiling: A Source Book for Health Care Administrators,
Neill F. Piland, Kerstin B. Lynam, Editors

Remaking Health Care in America: Building Organized Delivery Systems,
Stephen M. Shortell, Robin R. Gillies, David A. Anderson,
Karen Morgan Erickson, John B. Mitchell

The New Health Partners: Renewing the Leadership of Physician Practice,
Stephen E. Prather

Trust Matters: New Directions in Health Care Leadership,
Michael H. Annison, Dan S. Wilford

Health Care
in the New Millennium

Health Care in the New Millennium

Vision, Values, and Leadership

Ian Morrison

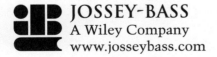

JOSSEY-BASS
A Wiley Company
www.josseybass.com

Published by

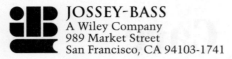

JOSSEY-BASS
A Wiley Company
989 Market Street
San Francisco, CA 94103-1741

www.josseybass.com

Jossey-Bass books and products are available through most bookstores. To contact Jossey-Bass directly, call (888) 378-2537, fax to (800) 605-2665, or visit our website at www.josseybass.com.

Substantial discounts on bulk quantities of Jossey-Bass books are available to corporations, professional associations, and other organizations. For details and discount information, contact the special sales department at Jossey-Bass.

We at Jossey-Bass strive to use the most environmentally sensitive paper stocks available to us. Our publications are printed on acid-free recycled stock whenever possible, and our paper always meets or exceeds minimum GPO and EPA requirements.

Library of Congress Cataloging-in-Publication Data

Morrison, J. Ian, date.
    Health care in the new millenium: vision, values, and leadership/Ian Morrison—1st ed.
      p. cm.—(The Jossey-Bass health care series)
    Includes bibliographical references and index.
    ISBN 0–7879–5115–3 (hardcover)
    ISBN 0–7879–6222–8 (paperback)
    1. Medical care—United States—Forecasting. I. Title. II. Series.
    [DNLM: 1. Delivery of Health Care—trends—United States. 2. Managed Care Programs—trends—United States. W 84 AA1 M72h 2000]
    RA395.A3 M675 2000
    362.1'0973—dc21   99-044361

FIRST EDITION
HB Printing   10 9 8 7 6 5 4
PB Printing   10 9 8 7 6 5 4

Contents

To Nora, David, Caitlin, and Bullet, with love

Preface

You've paid attention to keynote addresses on "The Future of Health Care." You have read the trade magazines and the popular press about the changing health care system. But you are still not sure what's really going on in health care. Maybe you are a little confused by the meteoric rise and apparent fall of managed care. Maybe you can't quite understand how the Clinton administration nearly implemented a national managed care plan in 1994 and then was trying to regulate managed care out of existence in 1999. Maybe you heard about vertically integrated systems as the wave of the future. Or disease-state management companies as the road ahead. Then there were hospitals owning doctors, hospitals owning other hospitals, or, God forbid, hospitals owning HMOs as the model for the future. Managed competition was going to be about a few large, vertically integrated HMOs like Kaiser competing head-to-head for patients. Never happened. Then the miracle of the managed care marketplace was supposed to keep costs low and quality high, making health insurance affordable for more people. How come premiums are rising again at 8 to 10 percent, and the number of uninsured is increasing? Then it was the consumer and the Internet, hand in hand solving the health care crisis as if by pixie dust. Confused?

The problem is that the future of health care really exists only on PowerPoint. We seem to jump from one future to another without implementing any of them. We talk about change, even though we do more wheel spinning than changing. We have lots of fabulous new medical technologies, but we also have the same old problems of cost, quality, access, and security of health benefits that we have worried about for the last thirty years. And they seem to be getting worse.

The reason we are dazed and confused about the future of health care is that we have never connected all the dots together. Health care is a product of the culture. Our vision of health care should reflect our values—not the values we would like to have but the ones we've got. Making that connection requires leadership. It requires leadership by politicians, by presidents, by policymakers, by entrepreneurs, by institutions (and their boards), by professionals, and by us as citizens, voters, and consumers. If we connect vision, values, and leadership, we can build a health care system that is at least coherent and sustainable. It might not be all that we want, but it would be better than what we have.

This book is a personal view of the future of health care, and, inevitably, it is shaped by my own values and background. I grew up in Glasgow, Scotland. In Glasgow, health care is a right; carrying a machine gun is a privilege. Somehow America got it the wrong way round. Ironically the only group of Americans with a right to health care are people in prison. Three strikes and you're covered.

I lived in Canada for almost ten years. I am married to a Canadian, and my son was born in Canada. Canadians are justly proud of their health system, a decent compromise between high-quality medicine and universal access—but a compromise that is culturally unavailable to Americans.

I studied health policy and economics in Canada, and my views have been affected by that experience and by my Scottish roots. I grew up in a place where doctors made house calls (and still do), and I lived, worked, and studied in a place where no one had to worry about access to a reasonable level of health care because of money.

For the last fifteen years I have lived and worked in California as a professional futurist (an oxymoron in and of itself). Although I have spent a good deal of time working outside of health care both in my work with the Institute for the Future and in independent practice, the majority of my time has been spent on my fascination with U.S. health care. I have been from the beginning intrigued, impressed, and appalled. I have been intrigued by the complexity of health care generally, but specifically in the United States with its myriad of institutions, actors, and organizational dynamics. I have been impressed with the dazzling brilliance of U.S. medicine at its technological best and by the enormous number of smart, dedicated people who work in all areas of U.S. health care. I have witnessed the enormous entrepreneurialism and business savvy of U.S. health care managers whether in the private, public, or independent sector. But I continue to be appalled that a country that is so rich, so smart, so motivated in so many ways can't offer all its residents access to health care.

As we enter a new millennium, the economy is in its longest-ever peacetime expansion, yet we see little or no prospect for major reform in U.S. health care. The industry is tired and battle weary. Leaders are not having fun. Doctors are cranky. Consumers reject both government solutions and market-based reforms. And there is widespread concern about the sustainability of the safety net and the economic viability of many organizations both public and private. America can do better.

This book, based on my twenty years of research and experience as a futurist, strategist, and consultant working with leadership groups in health care, was written to galvanize leadership. It is a humble attempt to provoke, inflame, excite, and insult the leaders in health care to stimulate them to try harder and build a better future.

We are not just one good *Health Affairs* article away from solving the problems of U.S. health care. If health care in the United States is going to be better, fairer, and more cost-effective, it will require leaders to step up to the challenges of change.

Managed care has been the default future for U.S. health care for almost thirty years. Unlike most countries, the United States does not want to run its system from the top down through government fiat. And managed care has been a uniquely American response. We need to build on what we have learned, but we also need to innovate beyond managed care.

Positive change is unlikely unless the health care system of the future moves to be responsive to consumers and creates an acceptable environment for providers in general and physicians in particular. Doctors are as depressed as their patients are about health care. Physicians too must step up the leadership and describe a better future, one that does not involve the return to some imagined golden age that never was.

Health care managers are tired of constant change. Our trade associations and leadership groups are trying valiantly to stimulate a battle-scarred group who have fallen prey to endless rounds of management faddism.

Health care in the future will reflect the evolution of U.S. culture and the U.S. economy. We live at a time of high uncertainty about the overall direction of U.S. society. Will we continue on a path of economic prosperity, or will the global economic turmoil catch up to the United States and force us to confront even tougher choices about the cost, quality, and accessibility of health care? Will we embrace the market even more, or will health care be a foundation of a new American focus on building a civil society?

Health care leaders cannot change the course of the global economy nor change the basic values of U.S. society. But they can innovate, build communities, develop outstanding institutions, and motivate and inspire their colleagues. Through leadership, health care can improve. Let's take on the leadership challenges and build a better health care system. I hope this book helps shed light on the challenges ahead.

Overview of the Contents

Chapter One explores the importance of values as a basic building block of policy and practice. Throughout American health care, the vision and values of various stakeholders are often at odds with one another. For example, the United States celebrates new medical technologies, but those same technologies are also a source of relentless cost pressures.

Chapter Two lays out the leadership challenges in health care for a wide variety of stakeholders. Throughout the health care system, leaders face important challenges, particularly in finding a new model for the health care system beyond the simplistic view of managed care.

Chapter Three describes the primary driving forces behind any future of health care. These driving forces—the coming public discontent with health care, the emergence of reluctantly empowered consumers, the continued effects of the managed care revolution, the fruits of innovation from investments in the new biology, the lack of an adequate information technology (IT) infrastructure despite the promise of the Internet, and the rediscovery of community—combine to create change. But the trajectory for U.S.

health care—the default future—isn't very pretty. It is one where more Americans are uninsured, where patients pay more and potentially get less, where large purchasers (both public and private) limit their own liability for health care, where managed care is defanged over quality (by regulations aimed at protecting consumer choice), where health care costs rise, and where Wall Street is disappointed with most health care services. Pharmaceuticals companies stand alone as being on a roll. But in pharmaceuticals, too, there is need for concern as the technological and economic success of the industry may lead to a backlash from the managed care industry or (more scary for the industry) through government price regulation.

Chapter Four describes five of the fundamental challenges of change in U.S. health care: the tension between health and health care; the search for a theoretical framework for health care—if not managed competition, then what?; the challenge of making community-based integrated systems work; the confusion over for-profit and not-for-profit health care; and the profound challenge of regional diversity in an enormous country.

Chapter Five describes how we got to managed care as the key instrument of both U.S. health care policy and the U.S. health care marketplace. It lays out the evolution of managed care and the key impediments to meaningful change.

Chapter Six places U.S. health care in a global context and shows that even though many countries around the globe share the common challenge of delivering high-quality health care at an acceptable cost, they are doing it in very different ways that reflect their culture and values. Although there are opportunities for countries to learn from one another, health care systems cannot be imported or exported whole cloth. The United States is on its own in forging a unique solution.

Chapter Seven highlights the unique role that purchasing plays in U.S. health care. The role of public and private purchasers who flex their muscle—the Big Ugly Buyers, as I have termed them—is a central one in health care reform. Medicare and Medicaid together account for a significant share of U.S. health care funding. The future of Medicare is the central question in contemporary U.S. health policy. Similarly, large employers played a significant part in creating the managed care revolution. But their role in the future will be less important as they pass the burden more to their employees and potentially leave the field altogether.

Chapter Eight explores the emerging consumerism in health care. Some affluent consumers are purchasing health care the same way they purchase other goods and services, by trading up to higher-quality services and brands with their own money. But even more consumers are reluctantly empowered; they are being asked by employers and government to take on more responsibility for payment and decision making in health care.

Chapter Nine assesses the current and future directions for health plans as they confront the challenges of a changing marketplace. Health plans are likely to default to one of three strategies: vertically integrating for value, as in the Kaiser model; becoming what I call a virtual single payer, which entails using contracting clout among large discounted fee-for-service provider networks as a way to deliver low cost and high choice of provider; and differentiating, which is based on a focus on the consumer, product differentiation, or distribution channel changes. There is precious little of the differentiation strategy among health plans.

Chapter Ten focuses on providers and the strategies available to them. Physicians need to change and to explore the broader possibilities of medical practice in the new millennium. Hospitals, too, need to confront a different future. Emerging strategies include developing horizontal cartels, creating local benevolent monopolists, and becoming focused specialty organizations. But hospitals and physicians are not alone in confronting change: academic medicine, long-term care, and the pharmaceutical industry each have important challenges ahead.

Chapter Eleven addresses the lack of strategy innovation among all constituents in health care. Drawing on Gary Hamel's insights about the role of innovation in the creation of strategy, the chapter focuses on ways health care organizations can improve their strategic thinking.

Chapter Twelve describes four alternate scenarios for health care that may evolve in the early part of the new millennium. The four scenarios highlight the uncertainties about sustained economic growth and the degree of civility in U.S. society. They describe alternate worlds for health care in which health care could be (1) locally focused, (2) reformed nationally, (3) mired in economic and social malaise, or (4) transformed in a manner similar to the transformation of financial services in a booming economy.

Chapter Thirteen concludes with some lessons about vision, values, and leadership. The bottom line: we need to be clear about values, we need to communicate across constituencies, we need to focus on getting physicians involved in change, we need to engage consumers honestly, and we need constantly to try to develop new and better visions for the future. Health care can be better when we imagine a better future.

September 1999   IAN MORRISON
Menlo Park, California

Acknowledgments

The health care field is complex, perhaps the most complex of any area of the economy. This book is an attempt at synthesis across the health care landscape. It is influenced by the training I received and the experiences I have had in health care in both Canada and the United States over the last twenty years. I am deeply grateful for the opportunity to work in health care, and I am indebted to the many individuals and organizations that I have had the privilege to work with over that period. The responsibility for errors, omissions, and insults is mine. What is written here should in no way reflect on the organizations with which I am affiliated, neither the Institute for the Future nor Andersen Consulting. This is an independent perspective on health care, and I take full responsibility for it.

I am particularly grateful to the following organizations and individuals. The Institute for the Future (IFTF) provided me an opportunity to work in the health care field with a wide variety of clients in the for-profit, nonprofit, and independent sectors. Through my involvement as adviser to the institute's project for the Robert Wood Johnson Foundation, I have had the opportunity to keep in touch with the fine work that IFTF does in the field of health care futures. Dr. Wendy Everett, director of IFTF's health care program, has built a great team.

Andersen Consulting has provided me an opportunity to chair a number of Health Futures Forums on the future of health care internationally, and this has given me insights into both the U.S. and the global health care scene. In particular I would like to thank Larry Leisure, Jim Hudak, David Rey, and Bob Rebitzer for sharing their perspectives on health care.

Over the last fifteen years I have had a partnership with Louis Harris and Associates, the nation's premier survey research firm in health care, and the Department of Health Policy and Management at Harvard University School of Public Health. Harris chairman Humphrey Taylor, president and CEO Bob Leitman, senior vice president Katherine Binns, and vice president Matthew Holt are wonderful colleagues and good friends. I am constantly stimulated by the new insights that Harris-Harvard research produces, and I have learned much about health care from each of them. Dr. Robert Blendon and Dr. Karen Donelan of the Harvard University School of Public Health are the premier scholars in the country in the area of public opinion in health care and its implications for the future of health policy and management. Bob Blendon was senior vice president at the Robert Wood Johnson Foundation and sponsor of a study in the early 1980s called Looking Ahead at American Health Care, a grant that brought me to join IFTF and subsequently lead IFTF's health care program. Both Bob and Karen have taught me much over the years.

Much of my recent work in health care has been in independent practice as adviser, author, consultant, moderator, and speaker. In particular, I would like to thank Kathryn Johnson and her colleagues at the Health Forum. I have greatly enjoyed my role as synthesizer at the Annual Health Forum Summit. I have learned much from the interactions with faculty and summit participants. In addition, earlier versions of chapters in this book have been published in what is now the *Health Forum Journal,* and I am grateful to the journal's editor, Elizabeth Zima, for her counsel and advice.

My thanks go to my literary agent, Rafe Sagalyn, for steering me through the publishing process once more, and to Jossey-Bass senior health editor Andy Pasternack and his wonderful staff for their enormous contributions.

My board relationships at Interim Services, Oceania, and the Health Research and Education Trust have given me an opportunity to learn about health care from new perspectives. I am deeply grateful to my fellow board members and to the CEOs of the organizations, Ray Marcy, Tom Durel, and Dr. Mary Pittman (respectively), for their insight, wisdom, and friendship.

I entered the health care field by accident. I was a geographer and urban planner who became hooked on health care. Dr. David Hardwick at the University of British Columbia, Canada, introduced me to the health care field and provides me to this day with important insights into the medical mind. Both David and his brother Dr. Walter Hardwick taught me much about synthesis across a wide range of policy and planning issues, for which I am very grateful. Dr. Robert Evans and Dr. Morris Barer have been important influences in helping me understand the health economics field from a non-U.S. perspective. The theoretical and applied lessons I learned from them in Canada have been invaluable in forecasting the strategic behavior of organizations in the United States. Indeed, I have often remarked that I combined Bob Evans's Economics 384 course and three jokes and turned it into a career.

To the hundreds of organizations and individuals in health care I have worked with over the last twenty years, I am deeply grateful for the opportunity to work with you.

Finally, to my family, thank you for your love and support. And Nora, you're right, a country as great as the United States should be able to provide health care coverage to everyone.

I. M.

Health Care
in the New Millennium

Chapter One

Health Care Vision and Values

The U.S. economy is on a roll, but the health care field is in the doldrums. Health care reform in Washington unraveled in the mid-1990s. The miracle of the managed care marketplace didn't really deliver. We seem to have run out of good ideas and are becoming increasingly vulnerable to half-baked or outright bad ideas. In Washington and the state capitols, the two principal policy objectives are to regulate managed care and to punish fraud and abuse by providers—both Band-Aids at best.

Health plans lost huge amounts of money in 1997 and 1998. Many hospitals that had been doing reasonably well started losing money in 1998, with more losses in 1999 in the wake of the Balanced Budget Act of 1997, which cut Medicare reimbursement rates for hospitals.

Although it often seems that the current problems we face in health care emerged overnight, they are the direct result of the accumulated policy decisions and market choices made over the last fifty years. Medicare and Medicaid were originally relatively small programs targeted to vulnerable groups; as the baby boomers age, these programs will become enormous entitlement programs funded by a shrinking number of workers. Employment-based insurance was a good idea when mainstream America worked for big, stable corporations; it seems less smart when people work as independent consultants or for Internet start-ups.

Health care is not in crisis, but we have lost the way forward, we have no clear vision of the future, and leaders seem tired. The big ideas of the past twenty years—managed competition, managed care, corporatization, and commmunity-based integration—have unraveled in implementation. The rise of consumerization and the Internet is now supposed to solve it all—not quite.

Health care is in need of renewal, reinvigoration, and leadership. The field desperately needs creativity and innovation, on the one hand, and pragmatic and long-overdue execution of well-established ideas, on the other.

Leadership, or more accurately the vacuum in leadership, is perhaps the single largest issue facing the health care system in the future. If meaningful change is going to occur in the next millennium, it's got to start sometime. The starting point is going to come from leadership inside the health care system, not necessarily from some brilliant new big idea from out of the blue. The leadership challenge starts with vision and values.

Vision and Values

Health care systems are the product of the culture. They are an organizational embodiment of societal values. The leadership challenge is to design health policy, build institutions, and manage care in a way that is consistent with our values. In fact, resolving the leadership challenges described in this book begins with values. Yet there is precious little discussion of values. Even during the health care reform debate of the early 1990s, values and principles were never really addressed. They were made manifest in the passive-aggressive sniping at the Clinton health plan proposal (the American Health Security Act) as being big-government, bureaucratic, or anti-American. Conversely, the Clinton plan tried to sneak through liberal values of social justice without clearly identifying them as such.

We are unlikely to make meaningful progress in building a better health care system unless we have more meaningful dialogue about values in our policymaking, in our organizations, and in our communities.

Global Health Care Values

Values are important determinants of health policy and health management. A good starting point in understanding the role of values is to compare the health care values of the United States with those of other countries. Most other developed countries, including most of Europe, Australia, and Japan, have relatively similar values with regard to health care despite the deep societal differences among these countries. Most countries hold the following values:

- *Universality.* Health care is universal. Everyone is included, even if the method of coverage may vary. At one extreme, universality is achieved by indirect means, such as mandatory coverage imposed by government but provided by individuals (as in Singapore) or by employers and labor groups (as in Germany). At the other extreme, universality is achieved in more direct form, as in the United Kingdom, where the National Health Service owns and operates a health care system that is available to all British residents.

- *Equity.* In many countries there is a sense that there should be equality before the health care system just as in equality before the law. Although this view is espoused most often and most loudly in Scandinavia and Canada, it also is a value that is held widely in Europe. The systems may not always deliver the same service to all residents or citizens, but equity is nevertheless a prevailing value in health care, if not always a specific policy goal.

- *Acceptance of the role of government.* Most health systems acknowledge that markets fail in health care and in health insurance and that this market failure creates a necessary and important role for government or government-like organizations. Not all German and Japanese sickness funds are government controlled, but they all behave in a highly coordinated fashion.

- *Skepticism about markets and competition.* Many countries are skeptical about markets and competition in health care, although this attitude is changing. In particular the World Bank, long perceived as being antimarket in the field of health care, has started to promote privatization and market mechanisms to energize health care. This move is partly a reaction against the way government central planners concentrate high-tech resources in the developing world.

- *Global budgets.* Most countries that have successfully contained costs have done so from the top down using global budgets. Although this approach may create microinefficiency, it has succeeded in containing the relative expansion of the health care sector with apparently no negative consequence to overall health status.

- *Rationing.* The consequence of global budgets is rationing. Here again, this value is not universally viewed as a negative. I grew up in postwar Britain, where the legacy of rationing was still evident. To the British, rationing is individual sacrifice for the common good, and it helped defeat the evils of Nazi Germany.

• *Technology assessment and innovation control.* A related but less extreme value is a belief in the assessment of technology and the management of innovation. Although this value may not be held by the population as a whole, it is a central value of many of the policymaking elites in such countries as Canada, the United Kingdom, and Scandinavia. In this model, the double-blind randomized trial is the gold standard, and relatively unproven technologies, such as fetal monitoring, are either not approved or not reimbursed because they fail to pass hurdles of both efficacy and cost-effectiveness.

U.S. Health Care Values

The United States holds a different set of values with regard to health care. In many cases, these values are diametrically opposed to the prevailing global values:

• *Pluralism and choice.* The United States values pluralism as both an end and a means. Choice is the surrogate for quality in U.S. health care; whether the scientific evidence supports this conclusion or not is irrelevant.

• *Individual accountability.* Americans value the freedom of the individual, and with those individual freedoms go responsibilities. In health care, we hear about the lack of individual accountability and responsibility for health with regard to such behaviors as the use of drugs, alcohol, and tobacco; overeating; and lack of exercise. At the extreme, individual responsibility is extended to cover the notion that individuals are responsible for their own health insurance. The argument is that if people choose to be uninsured, that's their choice and their problem.

• *Ambivalence toward government.* The American public is ambivalent toward governmental solutions. Typically, big government is portrayed as bad by members of both mainstream political parties. It is ironic that the two big-government programs of the century—Medicare and Social Security—remain the most politically popular and are stoutly defended by Republicans and Democrats alike.

- *Progress, innovation, and new technology.* America is the frontier. We embrace progress, innovation, and new technology. We want a cutting-edge health care system. And we place a continuing high priority on medical research and medical innovation of all types. Just look at our popular media, which daily celebrate medical miracles.
- *Volunteerism and communitarianism.* Americans are not uncaring. Volunteerism is a uniquely American value. Social welfare countries have high marginal tax rates; rich people give at the office, literally, so there is little interest in the United Way or its equivalent. The United States, like many other cultures, has strong elements of communitarianism, seen in many places: Southern black churches, barn-raising farming communities, or in whole states—Minnesota, Iowa, and Wisconsin.
- *Paranoia about monopoly.* Americans are paranoid about monopoly. If you have a big country and a small population, as in Canada or Australia, monopoly is less troubling. There is an argument that certain kinds of local nonprofit health care monopolies might not be such a bad thing, but it flies in the face of mainstream American concerns about monopoly. Ask Bill Gates.
- *Competition.* Americans like to compete even when it doesn't do us any good. In the United States, competition is an end, not just a means to an end. We like the process.

Consumerism and Net Culture

Two new values are coming to the fore both in the United States and around the world, although they are clearly more advanced in the United States:

- *Consumerism.* The rise of consumerism is part of a global value shift in health care. It reflects rising global education levels, rising incomes in the top tiers of global society, and increased sophistication in communication. The new consumers are emerging across the globe. They are demanding better customer service, they want to be involved in medical decision making, and they will reach out to alternative therapies as part of their medical care. The corollary of increased consumerism and segmentation in health care is tiering—a widening gap between rich and poor.

- *Net culture.* The Internet is feeding this consumerism and transforming it at the same time. The Net, unlike broadcast media, knows no international boundaries and opens up the possibility of both health care information exchange and electronic commerce (e-commerce) across national boundaries.

No Societal Consensus for Major Health Reform

A key impediment to major reform in the U.S. health system is the lack of common values. In contrast to other systems around the globe, there is no American consensus on such values as these:

- *Health care as a right.* Should health care be universally available to all citizens (and perhaps all residents)? (Slim majorities in surveys respond that health care is a right, but that is not the same as saying that a majority of voters support such a view or that a national political consensus exists to make health care a right; see *Health Affairs,* winter issue 1998.)
- *Equity.* Is the health care system based on the principle that everyone gets the same benefits, the same access, and the same quality of service?
- *Public administration.* Is the system a public service or a market good?

In most other countries, issues such as universality or equity or public dominance of the health care system are not equivocal. In Canada, for example, even the private sector holds values similar to those of the public at large. A strategic planning session was held in Montreal in 1997 with a series of leaders from the for-profit health care industry in Canada: private health insurers, pharmaceutical companies, and benefit consultants who organize the supplementary benefits in the Canadian health care system. These stakeholders could not foresee a Canadian system in which either the specifics of the Canada Health Act of 1984 or the basic tenets of the Canadian health care system that the act reinforced—universality, equity, and public administration—would be abandoned or substantially eroded. Rather, their vision was of identifying alternative ways in which the private sector could participate meaningfully in helping the mainstream medical system control costs and be more responsive to consumers.

In Canada, in Sweden, and in many other countries around the world, universality is not questioned. Similarly, the concept of equity (that is, the idea that the kind of health care system available to one group of the population should be identical to that received by people of very different economic circumstances) is accepted in many countries throughout Scandinavia as well as in Canada (although the inequities in Canada tend to be geographic rather than by income). For example, the Vancouver/Richmond Health Board in British Columbia stated the following as one of its eleven principles: "The framework for the delivery of health care will be based on the ideals of social justice and equitable access to service. (Equitable access refers to the removal of barriers to service delivery and decision-making about care for all segments of the population)."

In the United Kingdom, the vast majority of people—over 90 percent—use the National Health Service as the mainstream care provider and the only source of health insurance. Those who have supplementary insurance in the United Kingdom, approximately 10 percent of households, do not use that particular coverage to trade up in any meaningful sense to advanced health care services. The access to supplementary insurance allows them to jump the queue for more minor operations—varicose veins and so forth. Very few Britons are using their supplementary insurance to get cardiac surgery, for example, because there really are no parallel cardiac surgery facilities outside the National Health Service.

In most developed countries, health care is a right, and there is no equivocation. Access to some form of health care services is regarded as a right in almost all countries of the developed world and among the rapidly developing economies of Asia. Taiwan, for example, has recently instituted a system of universal coverage, albeit a program relatively basic in its scope.

In the United States, health care is not a right, and there is no societal or political consensus to make it so. The concept of equity is more appealing to Americans as a goal for justice (as in "justice for all") than it is for health care. There does appear to be consensus that the health care system should be tiered—that people should have the right to trade up with their own money. Polls also indicate that although Americans believe government should play an important role in helping the elderly and the poor get access to health care services, they fall far short of supporting a health care system run by government or paid for exclusively by government.

If we are to make meaningful progress in leadership in U.S. health care, then leaders must recognize these values as they exist, not as they might want them to be. As Bob Evans, the Canadian health economist, once said, "Americans are both a humane and brutal people." America wants a mixed public and private model. We want government to provide a safety net, but we also value pluralism and competition. We want a president who feels our pain and a Congress that does not spend any money relieving it. More specifically, Americans believe in floors and ceilings. We want a basic floor below which no American falls, and a ceiling—the right to use our own money to trade up to a nicer waiting room and better service. As Monty Python put it in the famous Piranha Brothers sketch: we want a system that is "cruel but fair."

The Crisis of Theory

Part of the current leadership problem in U.S. health care is that we have no operating theory for health policy or for market strategy. The default policy over the last twenty years has been the theory of managed competition promulgated by Alain Enthoven of Stanford University and by Paul Ellwood, founder of the Jackson Hole Group and widely regarded as the father of the modern HMO.

According to the theory of managed competition, sophisticated sponsors, such as large employers, assist cost-conscious consumers in selecting among competing health plans. Health plans—large vertically integrated entities like Kaiser Permanente—compete for consumers on the basis of cost and quality. Consumers select the plans once a year when they are well and live with the consequences when they are sick.

This theory has in fact been the prevailing vision of the future not only in the United States but also in many countries around the world, where there was significant interest in health reform on a managed competition model—for example, in Sweden, New Zealand, and the United Kingdom. Global interest in managed competition does not reflect a desire for wholesale replication of the U.S. health care system—"God forbid," as some of my colleagues abroad would say. Rather, this interest reflects an understanding that elements of privatization and competition might stimulate somewhat intransigent government-run health care services into being more responsive to a more affluent and sophisticated public and more accountable to the payers of the bill, be they consumers or government.

Managed competition was and is an appealing theory because it was a policy compromise that was consistent with many American values, such as competition, pluralism, individual accountability, and a limited role for government. In the United States, however, there has been a dramatic fall in managed competition as the basis for health care policy.

Managed competition was the operating principle behind the plan of California Health Insurance Commissioner John Garamendi in the late 1980s, an effort to reform California health care crafted by a coalition of health policymakers. The Garamendi plan became the base model for the Clinton health plan: the American Health Security Act. However, after health care czar Ira Magaziner and the Health Care Taskforce were finished, it became the grand unified field theory of health care. The unwieldy document was open to the ridicule of telegenic and articulate Republican scholars, such as Elizabeth McCaughey, a constitutional scholar at the Manhattan Institute. McCaughey rose to national political prominence (becoming New York's lieutenant governor) after she helped assassinate the Clinton health plan with a deft and well-researched little one-page editorial in the *New Republic* and numerous appearances on talk shows that pointed to the bureaucratic excesses of the Clinton proposal.

Enthoven and Ellwood never fully embraced the Clinton plan as their child. In fact, in the course of the unwieldy Clinton health plan policymaking process, both Ellwood and Enthoven were rudely dealt with by arrogant policy wonks who were dismissive of the professors' pleas for compromise with the private sector. Nevertheless, despite its lack of theoretical purity, the Clinton plan bore a very striking resemblance to managed competition.

Once the Clinton health plan was killed (or died under its own weight, depending on your perspective), a second era of managed competition emerged in the form of marketplace reform. In essence, the idea behind marketplace reform was that unregulated market competition—unmanaged competition if you like—would yield the same results as the more complete regulated form proposed by the Clintons. (It is somewhat ironic that when Enthoven and Ellwood first conceived of the notion of managed competition in the original paper by Enthoven, the proposed title was "Regulated Competition," which was an offensive oxymoron to the private sector. "Regulated" was changed to "Managed" to give it more appeal to the private sector.)

The notion of the health care marketplace as a better form of managed competition gained a lot of currency in 1995 and 1996. Health care cost increases slowed through the brutally competitive part of the underwriting cycle in the period 1995 to 1997. This was held up by many in the right wing as clear evidence that the market was working. But this was the era of what I call the Republican Paradox: the market is working, but managed care stinks.

Managed care contained costs, but it also became more unpopular with the public and the providers of health care during this period. Clearly a more competitive managed care marketplace had some effect on containing health care costs and certainly deserves significant credit for slowing the rate of growth in health care over this period. However, we gave far too much credit to the managed care marketplace for this effect and not enough credit to Hillary Clinton for scaring the bejeezus out of the U.S. health care industry, causing everybody to keep their heads down for two years in terms of both prices and utilization.

But the growing dissatisfaction with managed care coupled with the failure of some of the significant players in pure-market health care (Oxford Health Plans, Columbia/HCA, and Med-Partners-Mullikin being perhaps the most notable examples) led to the death of marketplace reform as the obvious theoretical answer for the future.

Marketplace managed competition died as the endgame as it became evident that competition had not permanently reduced health care cost inflation nor eliminated the inexorable rise of medical technology, the increased utilization and pricing of new pharmaceuticals, or the rise in medical utilization for visits, tests, and procedures. By 1998 it became increasingly evident that health care costs were on the rise again. Health premiums for employers began to rise, and managed care plans, instead of reaping enormous profits as they did by some analysts' estimation in the 1994 to 1996 period, saw their profits turn to losses in 1997 and 1998. If managed competition in pure theoretical form, in Clinton form, or in market form wasn't going to work, what was the theory for the future?

The Death of Big Ideas

Early in 1997, the managed care marketplace started to unravel as the clear winning theoretical formula for the future. The losses experienced by HMOs were spectacular. Perhaps the most spectacular of them all was Oxford Health Plans. Oxford lost over 75 percent of its market value in one day of trading. Oxford had done so much right with its consumer focus: they had reached out to yuppie clients and provided New Yorkers (the most difficult health care consumers on the planet) with an option to join managed care in a way that even New Yorkers could find acceptable. By signing up Park Avenue doctors, paying them reasonable rates, using creative utilization review and medical management, and selecting healthy New Yorkers in the first place, Oxford hoped that costs could be kept in line and that profits could be secured. Unfortunately, Oxford was challenged in a couple of minor ways. First, they couldn't pay claims, and, second, they couldn't do medical management very well. These are not small challenges if you are an HMO.

Others in the managed care marketplace who were supposed to be pioneers and winners of the future, such as the physician practice management (PPM) companies, also have been spectacular in their demise. They have been exposed as Ponzi schemes in which sustained profitability seems unlikely.

In the search for the next big idea, many in the private sector, in particular, latched on to consumerism and consumer centricity. Although it is undeniable that part of the future of American health care will involve being more responsive to increasingly sophisticated consumers in terms of customer service, customer involvement in decision making, and speed and flexibility in health care delivery, it would be wrong to assume that we are in any way close to having a purely consumerist marketplace in which gleeful consumers trade up and select among competing institutions with their own money. It is a neat conception but is grossly inaccurate because most Americans are not gleeful consumers of health care now, nor will they be in the future. Rather, what we're seeing is a rise of consumerism driven more by a willingness, however reluctant, to pay more to get what households believe is a reasonable value from an unresponsive and badly organized health care system.

There are a number of undeniable signs of consumerism in health care. First is the rise of alternative medicine. Although this trend has been amplified by the Food and Drug Administration's opening the floodgates for the approval of herbal remedies, the growth in alternative therapies is clearly an attempt by consumers to state their preferences with regard to health care and in some way show their discontent with the lack of responsiveness of mainstream medicine. Consumers see chiropractors, acupuncturists, and herbal therapists as providing useful benefits even if these therapies are not as scientifically rigorous as one would like (although I have pointed out to some of my medical colleagues that it is important for them not to get too prissy on this issue, considering there is not much science behind most mainstream medical therapies either).

The second undeniable sign of rising consumer preference is that consumers have been empowered, *empowered* being largely a code word for "You're on your own, pal." They have been empowered by the massive shift from defined benefit to defined contribution. (Defined-benefit health plans, like defined-benefit pensions, specify a schedule of benefits. A defined-contribution plan specifies only the amount that the employer or sponsor is prepared to contribute to secure the benefit.)

Consumers are voting with their feet and are being asked to pay more for health care, and to be responsible in the future for both selecting health plans and paying for their health care. This shift from defined benefit to defined contribution is pervasive and applies to both the public and private sectors. State government health benefit plans, federal government plans (the Federal

Employees Health Benefits Program), and large corporations (such as Xerox, General Electric, and Hewlett-Packard) have all moved toward a defined-contribution model. But this model also applies to Medicare and Medicaid, in which choice and selection are becoming much more prevalent. The shift from defined benefit to defined contribution is not in a pure form in which employees are given a voucher for a fixed amount of money. Rather, the sense is growing among employees and the Medicare program that health plan beneficiaries will have to pay a larger percentage of health premiums in the future. Consumerism, although a major trend, is not a wholesale solution.

The last new big idea is related to consumerism: the Internet. Somehow it is felt that health care can be increasingly delivered over the Internet. In *The Second Curve,* I wrote that the health system of the future would find its true Second Curve—the new way of doing business—only if it incorporated new technology, such as the Internet, and served sophisticated new consumers more appropriately. I still hold that to be the case, but it is important to emphasize that while e-commerce offers exciting new opportunities, not everything can be put on the Net, as we will discuss in more depth in Chapter Ten.

Chapter Two

Health Care Leadership Challenges

Overall, the health system is desperately in need of an underlying set of values and a set of new ideas. A successful U.S. health system of the future will incorporate both floors and ceilings. In other words, Americans want a basic floor below which no American falls. This really speaks to the American sense of fairness. But Americans also want a set of ceilings—the right to trade up with their own money—because this approach respects the American pursuit of individualism, pluralism, and the right to purchase superior quality with earned income.

From a political perspective, however, it is difficult to see how these desires and these fundamental values can be reconciled. A U.S. electorate that is socially liberal and fiscally conservative seeks consistently to split the political baby by electing a Congress and an executive branch from opposing parties. It is therefore likely that considerable political leadership will be required to broker the compromise between these disparate underlying values in any health system of the future. But meaningful change in health care will require leadership from many stakeholders both inside and outside health care. It is to these leadership challenges that we now turn.

Political Leadership Challenges in Health Care

The politics of health care are the subject of innumerable books and scholarly articles, and it is not my purpose here to replay the political leadership issues involved in the transformation of health care. But as we analyze leadership and the absence of leadership in health care, it is important to look at the political landscape. The greatest historical example of political leadership in American health care was the Great Society legislation of the 1960s, which created Medicare and Medicaid. This legislation solved difficult problems. A huge historical opportunity to have more sweeping reform was not blown by trying to reach too far and extend government-sponsored coverage to all Americans. Although the resulting compromise planted the seeds for huge cost escalation through the 1970s and 1980s, Medicare and Medicaid at least provided security for the most vulnerable groups in society. In the Clinton health plan debate, by reaching too far we ended up going backward rather than forward. Some may argue that a more circumspect, humble, and limited health reform program would have put us in a better position today than the bold policy initiative attempted by the Clintons. Whether that is true or not, the attempted reform has left us with a less ambitious policy and political process for health care than we had prior to the Clintons' bold plans. There are no brownie points in health policy anymore. The political rewards for promoting sweeping health reform do not justify the risks.

Big health reform, on the Clinton model, requires a political consensus that sweeping changes are necessary. It is tough to whip up the euphoria of an entire nation more than once a decade on the same issue. The Democrats' default health agenda is to regulate HMOs, to preserve Medicare in its current form, and to make minor expansions in coverage for long-term care—not to make sweeping improvements in coverage for the forty-three million or more uninsured.

This more restricted set of political options results from Republican indifference meeting Democratic incrementalism. (Incrementalism at its worst is going from one bad idea to another bad idea; at its best, it is the taking of measured steps toward a broader, laudable goal—what I would call *strategic incrementalism*). Republicans, particularly the new crop who entered in 1994, do not care about the health care issue. We have a Republican party with little interest in health care and a Democratic party with no new ideas. The Democrats have backed off from their health reform positions of earlier decades, when they seriously pursued universality—at least for the elderly and the poor—and the Medicare and Medic-

aid programs made that pursuit manifest. Since that time, successive generations of Democrats have backed away from universality,
and the current debate centers more on regulating managed care
than on making meaningful expansions in coverage.

Medicare is a central policy issue for both parties because of
the political power of the elderly. The revival of Clinton's political
fortunes in 1996 was in no small part due to his casting the Republicans as undoing Medicare and himself as its stout defender. However, the Medicare debate as it ensued through at least the early
part of 1999 is a political football game fought on a very narrow
playing field. The fight is about small changes in premiums and
copays when the arguments should be about the sustainability of
the program once the baby boom really hits the wall in 2020.

It is possible that Congress will enact Medicare reform that will
bring the program closer to the Federal Employees Health Benefits Program. This reform would signal a shift from a defined-
benefit model for Medicare to one of defined contribution.

A further problem with the current mode of political incrementalism is that, however well meaning, the initiatives taken by
Congress and state legislatures in the 1990s to ameliorate the
plight of the uninsured and underinsured have often led to worse
rather than better coverage. For example, the well-meaning legislation in California on rate regulation of small-group insurance has
probably, if truth be known, led to increases rather than decreases
in the number of uninsured by raising the price of the average policy for those small businesses. Similarly, the proposals by the Clinton administration to make Medicare coverage available to the
fifty-five-year-old to sixty-four-year-old would, if implemented, probably lead to an unraveling of existing coverage by employers for
that age group.

Finally, in terms of the political leadership landscape, there is
a dearth of outrage about the uninsured. William Bennett's book
about the faults of the Clinton administration, *The Death of Outrage*,
had the right title but the wrong focus. The outrage that seems to
be missing in health care is around the question of the uninsured.
By 1997 there were 43.1 million uninsured in the United States and
no serious discussion at the policy level about addressing the issue.
Further, the rise in the number of uninsured is occurring at the
height of the longest-running economic expansion in a generation

and the lowest unemployment rate in decades. Simultaneously, employer-based coverage has eroded. The staggering tragedy in all of this is that a significant proportion—some 25 percent of these uninsured people—are children. Despite recent advances in coverage for kids in the so-called Kiddie Care legislation of 1998 (providing federal government funding to expand coverage for children in poverty), very few states have actually put in place meaningful programs that have addressed the needs of uninsured children. Children just don't seem to provoke the same level of outrage.

If we are to make meaningful progress in the politics of health care, we need to identify

- A framework for strategic incrementalism that leads toward the broader policy goal of sustainable universal coverage.
- Logical and consistent reform for the Medicare system that does not simply shore up the existing program but looks out to the sustainability of the program when the median baby boomers become eligible in the 2020s.
- A set of policies that can bring disparate values and disparate interests together. For example, we value technological innovation and we value affordability of pharmaceuticals and new medical technology; can we have both?

Leadership Challenges for Managed Care

Managed care, broadly defined, is now the mainstream of American health care. We have looked to managed care to lead us into the future, and we may have asked too much of it. For-profit HMOs have struggled because they were not equipped to lead, at least from a policy point of view. Alan Hoops, the CEO of PacifiCare, the leading managed care plan in the Medicare field, has often remarked that the traditional indemnity health insurance industry died too early. His argument is that in a very short period of time, for-profit managed care was thrust into the limelight as the leader of an entire health care industry rather than allowed to remain the loyal opposition—an alternative to mainstream health insurance. Managed care did indeed succeed in killing the traditional indemnity health insurance business; such titans as Metropolitan Life,

Travelers, and Prudential have all exited the business. However, the bitter irony for the managed care innovators (both for-profit and nonprofit) is that managed care in the United States is still largely discounted fee for service, not all that different from the products their now-dead rivals offered in the late 1980s.

Managed Care: Dazed, Demonized, and Confused

Managed care leaders suffer from what we might call the Wizard of Oz effect. When you get to know managed care leaders and pull back the curtain, you find frightened, middle-aged white guys who are making it up as they go along. Finding a sustainable business model in an era when then industry is unpopular is the key leadership challenge for managed care. Managed care leaders are often put in difficult positions, not only because managed care has become the mainstream of health policy, but also because they have suffered financial, organizational, and public relations losses. Even the managed care pioneers, the not-for-profit integrated HMOs, such as the Kaiser Foundation Health Plan and the Henry Ford Health System in Detroit—well-run, respected organizations—have experienced significant financial difficulty in the late 1990s. In particular, Kaiser lost almost $300 million in each of two years, 1997 and 1998. Kaiser returned to profitability in 1999, but this does not make up for the whittling away of a significant part of its accumulated surplus over the last fifty years.

Most managed care plans experienced financial misfortune in the late 1990s. First, the consumer backlash caused managed care plans to broaden their networks in the name of choice, thereby weakening contracting clout and utilization controls. Second, most HMOs experienced tremendous increases in pharmaceutical costs. Third, medical innovation led to related increases in utilization levels and intensity of servicing that continue to escalate despite the best efforts of managed care. Some of the leaders in the private sector of managed care, whether it be Oxford Health Plans or Prudential Insurance, have experienced spectacular failure.

Those managed care companies that are flourishing are doing so as "virtual single payers"—that is, such plans as WellPoint, Anthem, Highmark, and some of the other well-positioned, highly penetrated Blue Cross–Blue Shield for-profit conversions wield such market clout that they're able to price their services in a competitive way and are able to extract significant discounts from providers. If you own 30 percent of somebody's business, you have a very different conversation with him or her than if you own 3 percent of the business. In addition, because of their market clout, they can contract with a broad network of providers, which enables them to offer a wide choice of physicians—an important quality indicator.

At the national level, United HealthCare has pursued a similar strategy, entering markets where there is little or no managed care and reaching significant penetration in those markets so as to become the default managed care monopolist or oligopolist.

Similarly, among the national insurers, Aetna U.S. Healthcare gobbled up Prudential's health insurance business shortly after it had digested New York Life's NYLCare, prompting Edward Hanway, president of rival Cigna Healthcare, to remark in the *New York Times* that "size matters." For example, postmerger Aetna has almost 25 percent of the Dallas market; in 1988, national health insurers like Aetna were lucky if they had 4 percent in any metropolitan area.

Consolidation and concentration of purchasing power in a few select markets have proven to be perhaps the most robust strategy for managed care plans. In a five-year period, a dozen health care companies have been scooped up by six survivors: Aetna U.S. Healthcare, Cigna, United HealthCare, Foundation Health Systems, PacifiCare, and WellPoint Health Networks. Foundation Health Systems, and PacifiCare may not remain independent for long.

In contrast, those companies that have tried to focus on broad national market share by serving big brand-name national employers without local concentration of firepower have ended up going the way of the dodo bird. Metropolitan and Travelers were early victims of this strategy. That is why the single remaining players from the old-line health insurance industry, Aetna U.S. Healthcare and Cigna, must continue to consolidate their positions by adding and acquiring new blocks of business to reach significant local market dominance over the provider sector.

If finding a sustainable business strategy is the primary leadership challenge of managed care, the other significant leadership challenge facing the managed care industry is to deliver on its original promise of managing medical care. There is a legitimate role for managed care (whether for-profit or not-for-profit) as rationer in a country that does not believe in government. But if managed care is to provide leadership in transforming the utilization of services in the medical care system, it will have to make two important investments. First is investment in the *intellectual infrastructure* of medical management, to ensure that health services are used cost-effectively: investment in creating practice guidelines and drug formularies, improving quality assurance, and conducting research in technology assessment. If there is a legitimate managed care payoff, it is in the form of medical management. But improved medical management in turn requires a second form of investment: in the *information infrastructure* necessary to manage medical care. There has been an astonishing lack of change in the information infrastructure, not so much in the back office of managed care plans but in the clinical activities of physicians, where there is still a pitiful lack of clinical usage of information systems in the practice of medicine. Because many of the insurers are still burdened by steam-driven legacy systems, there is no clear consensus on what the future information infrastructure for health care should look like. Kaiser and a few of the other nonprofit integrated health care systems stand alone in making a $1 billion-plus commitment to upgrading the information infrastructure for clinical medicine.

Managed care is flailing around try to find a new future. These are the big leadership questions:

- Can Kaiser and the other vertically integrated health plans reassert their preeminence as leaders in innovation in health care delivery and in delivering both quality and value? And will the new consumer be convinced?
- Is the strategy of health plan consolidation sustainable? Will the virtual single payers own the future?
- Will innovators emerge in the managed care business, and will they be rewarded?
- Can managed care organizations overcome their negative image with the public and with physicians?

Leadership Challenges for
Hospitals and Health Systems

The leadership of the hospital industry is under stress partly
because of the diversity of circumstances facing hospitals. Hospitals find themselves in three very different categories of financial
success. First, there are the basket-case institutions that are held
together by bailing wire and disproportionate share funding. These
hospitals, often in the inner city, are in deep financial trouble
largely because of their heavy loads of uncompensated care, their
heavy Medicaid roles, and their significant uninsured populations
whom they are obligated to serve because of mission or mandate
from local or state governments. These organizations, the safety-
net providers, have teetered on the brink for many years. Some of
them are so centrally important to the poor of their communities
that they simply cannot go under for fear of overwhelming the for-
profit and other more mainstream providers with large numbers
of patients to look after. And so it is in everybody's interest in the
health system to ensure that they do not go under entirely. These
organizations receive disproportionate share funding (so-called
Dish payments) from the Health Care Financing Administration
(HCFA) to compensate for their burden of uncompensated
patients.

A second group of institutions (mostly nonprofit but including
almost all the for-profits) are teetering on the edge. In the mid-
1990s these organizations were doing quite well. They were dam-
aged but not destroyed by managed care. Indeed, their success in
the mid-1990s can be attributed to their fear that they would be
overwhelmed by capitation: they downsized and rightsized in
preparation for capitated reimbursement that never came, and by
so doing they improved their bottom line. This group of hospitals
is also the group that experimented on the edge of many innovations, including physician-hospital organizations (PHOs) and
provider-sponsored networks (PSNs). In the late 1990s, this mid-
dle-third group of institutions are surviving if not thriving. But they
became vulnerable to the reductions in funding of the Balanced
Budget Act of 1997, which started to erode Medicare margins once
again. This erosion, in combination with continued penetration of

managed care programs, is likely to put these institutions and their leadership under significant financial pressure through the first few years of the millennium.

The final third of hospitals are monopolists and loving it. These organizations tend to be located in the affluent suburbs of major metropolitan areas or in smaller towns or more rural locations with low unemployment and no significant Medicaid population in their community. Usually these are community-based, independent not-for-profit hospitals that also tend to be in states where there is not a significant penetration of Medicare risk (capitation payments for Medicare programs). Good examples of these organizations are Waukesha Hospital in Wisconsin, Lake County Hospital outside Cleveland, Washington County Hospital outside Baltimore, and Rush Copley Hospital on the west side of Chicago. Operating margins in these top-tier financial performers often exceed 10 percent—more than twice the national average in a good year. These are well-run organizations, passionately focused on their local community and capable of defending against incursion by either for-profit competitors or managed care organizations that would want to radically alter their patient base, particularly their Medicare patient base.

There is a profound leadership tension in American hospitals between CEOs' desire to do the right thing in terms of making their institutions more focused on the broader health of the community, on the one hand, and the need to ensure their institutions' survival, on the other. Most hospitals are still largely paid on a per diem basis or on the basis of the diagnosis-related group (DRG); that is, for inpatient services (and increasingly for outpatient services as well) the hospital is paid a standard fee for a particular diagnosis regardless of how long the patient stays in the hospital or how low or high the true cost of care. Most hospitals are DRG factories dependent on DRG funding from Medicare and from commercial insurers as the core of their reimbursement.

It is a myth that hospitals are increasingly capitated; in fact, very few hospitals receive global capitated payments. Capitation seems to be stalling rather than proliferating. By the end of 1998, the HCFA had received only three applications for PSN status. Hospital-based HMOs tend not to be particularly profitable, and most of them have been started as side bets by hospitals to protect themselves against the threat of market incursion from aggressive for-profit HMO competitors. They are conceived more as income-support schemes for providers rather than as meaningful managed care initiatives that change how care is delivered.

The profound tension in the hospital industry is also reflected in its trade association—the American Hospital Association (AHA). The AHA is way ahead of its constituency in terms of its strategic focus on healthier communities. Most local community hospitals that preach in their mission statements their interest in creating healthier communities are actually more keenly interested in their institutional survival. This focus on financial survival makes hospitals more centrally concerned about DRG rate levels and the generosity of reimbursement from managed care for a particular new technology than about the broader determinants of health, such as income and education.

The AHA and other trade groups in the hospital industry should be applauded for their leadership in trying to bring a reluctant sick-care industry closer to understanding and engaging in the determinants of health. But hospitals are the largest employers in most communities in America and one of the only large employers immune to global competition. Hospitals are both a community resource for medical care and a key employer. Perhaps it is ultimately most important to the community's health that the hospital focus on being around to fulfill those roles. Yet hospitals can provide leadership, focus, and support for other community-based organizations and for local government and development agencies to help those groups have an impact on the true determinants of health.

Hospitals need to do the following:

- Reconcile whether they are improving the health of their communities or just delivering sick care.
- Identify, as a group, public policy positions that make sense for all hospitals. There is the tyranny of the mean, in that the circumstances of the "arithmetic average hospital" do not reflect the experiences of any of them. Hospitals are either doing well or doing badly.

Leadership Challenges for Physicians

Doctors used to be the kings of the hill; now they are treated like pages. Physicians have been the least led over the last decade and the group most in need of leadership. As the new millennium dawns, who speaks for doctors? The American Medical Association (AMA) has seen continued erosion in its membership, and there is frustration on the part of physicians generally that the AMA does not serve and does not speak for all doctors.

Specialty societies similarly are struggling to speak for their physicians, many of whom are spread not only across the diverse regions of the country but also across the diverse circumstances of hospitals and managed care markets that we highlight in this book.

Traditional large group practices that are part of large HMOs such as the nine-thousand-physician Kaiser Permanente Medical Group have experienced the strains and pressures of a changing managed care marketplace as its long-time partner, Kaiser Foundation Health Plan, faced intense competition from other models. Many of the other independent large-group practices in California, such as Mullikin and Health Partners in Los Angeles, have struggled in recent years as their HMO partners have consolidated and as premiums have been stagnant.

Independent practice associations (IPAs) have often been no more than side bets for doctors, with physicians joining multiple IPAs as a means of accessing managed care patients. Most doctors do not have much faith in or loyalty to any particular IPA.

PPM companies (corporations who acquired physicians' practices, both large groups and small independents, claiming they could bring economies of scale to medical groups) and other for-profit organizations of physicians have had spectacular declines in the late 1990s. Although these organizations had the potential to become the equivalent of a private sector union for doctors, their demise really speaks to the inability of physicians to organize.

The recent interest in physician unionization reflects the frustration of America's doctors. But remember that this is not unionization in the traditional sense. Doctors do not want to become employees, join together and hold hands and sing "We shall overcome." What they want is a right to have countervailing monopoly bargaining power with HMOs while preserving their independence.

Medicine needs leadership. The terms *physician leaders* and *physician managers* are in many cases oxymorons. Richard Smith, the editor of the *British Medical Journal,* has an eloquent speech that he gives on physician leadership. To paraphrase his point: doctors deliberately elect leaders who nobody would want to follow so they can passive-aggressively undermine those leaders when they don't like their solutions. As one dean of a notable medical school noted, "I do OK in the meetings. It's in the corridors that I get killed." This points to the fact that physicians tend to be quietly acquiescent in management discussions but have an uncanny ability to undermine decisions taken in a group in their subsequent private conversations with their colleagues in the hospital corridors, physicians lounges, or operating rooms, not to mention the golf course (although physicians' golf handicaps must have suffered mightily in the last five years as the vagaries of managed care have required most doctors to work harder, spend more time on administration, and receive less income overall).

It is true that physicians are grouping together, huddling together for warmth as it were, in group practice or as employees of larger entities, trying in some way to get economies of scale in a business that really doesn't have any. The Medical Group Management Association is one of the key trade associations for group practice; their data indicate that larger group practices have a higher share of overhead going toward administration than do smaller groups. This is part of the reason why PPM companies never really made any money: there really aren't any inherent economies of scale in group practice.

Even the most pioneering physician leaders in health care, leaders of the capitated group practices of Southern California (such as Dr. Bob Margolis of Health Partners in Los Angeles), have become not the leading edge but the bleeding edge of medicine. Only a few short years ago, these capitated medical groups were the wave of the future because they accepted risk on a per member per month basis for all health care services. But leaders of these organizations are frustrated by HMOs who have ground down their remuneration, by pharmaceutical companies who have detailed around them, by employers who have opted for point-of-service plans that undermine these leaders' ability to manage referrals out-side their group, and by patients who confuse choice with quality. This situation leaves leaders in the capitated group setting with ever more difficult challenges. If PPM companies don't present the leadership for the future, if the AMA doesn't present the leader-ship, if capitated group practice doesn't present the leadership for the future, where can physicians expect to end up?

Doctors need to consider their future, because if they do not help develop some new visions for the future, if they do not show some leadership, then they can look forward to a future in which their circumstances are akin to those of physicians in Germany and Canada: they will be trapped in what I call the hamster model of reimbursement.

Doctors in Canada and Germany are like hamsters on a tread-mill. They must operate under a fixed sectoral budget (in a province, in the case of Canada) for all physician services, and under a standardized fixed-fee schedule established by government negotiation with physicians. Each physician tries to earn his or her own target income by providing more and more services, but as the utilization of the service goes up in total and exceeds the pre-set total budget for all physicians, so the fee for each service goes down. Like frantic hamsters, the physicians accelerate ever quicker around the little wheel trying to get to their individual target incomes, but in an effort to maximize their own incomes by pro-viding more service, they end up lowering the price for all physi-cians. In Canada, in certain provinces, such as British Columbia, the price decline is reinforced by absolute dollar limits on total income. Once physicians' total billings reach a preset limit, they will not be reimbursed for any subsequent services delivered in that period (usually a quarter). This causes physicians to take what is euphemistically called reduced activity days (RADs). In other words, there is little or no incentive for physicians to keep their practice doors open after they have achieved a certain amount of billing, which is precisely the intent of the reimbursement scheme. This reimbursement policy recognizes that although physician net income is but 10 percent of the total costs of care, doctors' activity and decisions are responsible for the vast majority of the remain-der. It's not the income of doctors that is the main reason for increasing health care costs. The main reason is the economic havoc doctors wreak trying to achieve that income in a fee-for-service system by providing health services that incur further costs in terms of drugs, surgery, and hospital utilization.

In an environment where HMOs are increasingly behaving as virtual single payers, U.S. doctors need to envision a better future than one of being a hamster on a treadmill—a future that does not involve a return to 1975 or some other imagined past.

Doctors need to help develop a future that

- Moves beyond a vision of the good old days when doctors were free to practice as they saw fit, charge what they wanted (so-called reasonable and customary charges), and not be accountable for either total cost or quality of care.
- Incorporates new models of organization and reimbursement more fitting for an age in which responsiveness to customers as well as technical excellence are valued.
- Is acceptable to the profession. Physicians are very upset. A health care system in which doctors are alienated and depressed is not a sustainable one.

Leadership Challenges for the Pharmaceutical and Medical Technology Industry

The pharmaceutical industry is on a roll. It is producing new products based on new technologies and getting faster approval for those new products. It is reaping the fruits of innovation and its investment in R&D, which was escalated significantly through the 1980s and early 1990s. Many of the leading companies—Pfizer, Glaxo-Wellcome, and Bristol-Myers Squibb—have invested significantly in their R&D and have not been sidetracked by pharmacy benefit management companies (PBMs, organizations that manage the drug benefit on behalf of employers) or by forays into managed care activities and ownership. They have focused specifically on what they do best: conduct R&D to produce new blockbuster drugs, price those drugs at extremely high levels, and promote those drugs to the profession and to the consumer. There is an aura of "you can't touch us" surrounding the industry right now.

Pharmaceutical companies have gone over the heads of managed care organizations and straight to consumers and physicians.

Direct-to-consumer marketing increased 30 percent in 1998 alone. Through TV, magazine, and newspaper advertising, pharmaceutical companies are taking their message directly to the public. If it weren't for pharmaceutical advertising supplements, *Newsweek* would be only three pages long. Similarly, pharmaceutical companies have focused on "detailing" physicians very aggressively (that is, promoting products through sales calls to doctors to provide information and free samples). Pfizer alone has forty-five hundred people in its sales force. Bristol-Myers Squibb and Hoffman–La Roche, for example, added over one thousand salespeople over the last couple of years. Drug companies know that putting sophisticated detailing teams in the field to promote their products to doctors makes a difference in prescribing behavior. Doctors may find this offensive, but detailing works.

Pharmaceutical companies have succeeded in coping with formularies imposed by managed care organizations and Medicaid. They have ensured that they are on the formulary by providing the managed care organizations with sophisticated pharmaco-economic rationales for the inclusion of their product. And if that approach doesn't work, they go over the heads of those managed care organizations to the CEOs of the health plans or to attorney generals, to the media, or to the Medicaid commissions to ensure that their drug is included.

The combination of sophisticated managed care marketing with direct-to-consumer advertising and physician detailing has stimulated both the use and costs of pharmaceuticals for managed care plans and, in so doing, is killing the managed care industry. Several CEOs of health care plans in California have privately pointed to the fact that sometime between 2000 and 2002, depending on the commercial HMO product, drug costs within an HMO, at around $22 per member per month, will exceed inpatient hospital costs.

In a recent survey of pharmaceutical industry executives, Louis Harris and Associates found that the pharmaceutical industry's plan for the future was for more of the same. Expect even more focus on R&D and drug development, more focus on direct consumer advertising, and more focus on the detailing of physicians. The executives surveyed anticipate that doing more of the same will result in continued escalation in profit for the industry.

The leadership challenge for the pharmaceutical industry is to continue its innovation and enormous financial success without alienating

- A struggling managed care industry, which places part of the blame for its financial problems on pharmaceutical costs that are growing by 15 to 20 percent annually.
- Consumers, who will have to pay more for drugs out of pocket as their drug coverage erodes and their copayments rise from $5 to as much as $50.
- Physicians and other providers, to whom the industry is aggressively promoting its products; it is also causing significant financial hardship for providers, as a higher share of costs going to pharmaceuticals means less money for providers, both hospitals and physicians.
- Government, which will eventually respond to the antipharmaceutical backlash from health plans and providers and from patients—the elderly in particular—as they pay higher out-of-pocket costs. Pharmaceuticals could become a key government target for price and coverage reforms.

Leadership Challenges for Public Health and the Safety-Net Providers

The public health community and the safety-net providers—county health departments and the large inner-city hospitals—are different from mainstream community health care, almost isolated. Part of the isolation is self-induced. The public health and safety-net community can be incredibly self-righteous about having a monopoly on compassion for the poor. This self-righteousness extends to an antagonism toward the medical model; toward the not-for-profit health care sector's focus on more affluent, well-insured consumers; and particularly toward the pharmaceutical and managed care industries and their for-profit orientation. This antagonism has probably led to a lack of integration and engagement with the broader health care system and to an unwillingness to embrace managed care principles, tools, and activities.

Leaders in the field, such as Roz Lasker of the New York Academy of Medicine, point to the need for public health to integrate more closely with medicine and managed care. But public health is torn between being an advocate for health and an evaluator of health services for the whole community, on the one hand, and being the safety-net provider for one group of the population, on the other.

Most safety-net providers tend to be hospital centered and institutionally focused. Their default strategy is to provide as much primary care service as they can afford with the categorical funding they receive and provide hospital care for the impoverished acutely ill. An open and overcrowded emergency room becomes a surrogate for systematic health services for the poor and uninsured.

The tension between being a public health advocate and being a safety-net provider overwhelms the leadership in the public health community: If they don't provide services to the disadvantaged, who will? It is important to note that these people have dedicated their careers, and their lives in many instances, to serving people in need. The risk of burnout for this leadership group is extreme. When the next recession comes, this group could burn out for good. Public health leadership could be stretched to the breaking point in the next recession because we have cut health care coverage and welfare at the height of the economic expansion. Even if the economic good times do extend well into the new millennium, as they may, there will be a lack of major policy action during these economic good times. We will have economic surpluses but no political willingness to use those surpluses to make meaningful changes in the safety net for working-class Americans, either through coverage expansion or major investment in safety-net institutions.

If the next recession is as ugly as one might imagine, it is not inconceivable that there might be sixty million uninsured. Such a recession could occur just when the public health leadership is aging and the key public health institutions are financially vulnerable and sorely in need of reinvigoration. This could be the recipe for disaster: these institutions could collapse permanently. Some might argue that such a collapse may be the stimulus for more meaningful global reform. Looking at history, however, we see the political and economic conundrum that public support for major change in coverage is greatest in times of economic crisis, precisely the time when the country has the least ability to pay for such change. That is why this current economic prosperity presents a unique opportunity, because we do have economic prosperity at the same time that we have a socially vulnerable middle class and forty-three million uninsured. Yet we do not seem likely to make sweeping expansions in coverage.

The public health community needs to decide

- Whether it is going to participate in the mainstream of medical care in general and managed care in particular, or is going to remain off at the side as a critic of U.S. health care
- Whether it is an evaluator of health services and advocate for health improvement, or the provider of last resort
- How to incorporate the ideas of population health into the mainstream political agenda for health care without sounding too much like socialism for the average American to handle

Leadership Challenges for Foundations

Foundations historically have played a major leadership role in the U.S. health care system. They have led by leveraging their limited financial resources to demonstrate best practices (in the case of clinical reform) or to stimulate the quality of medical care through investment in teaching and research programs. Thus foundations have had a major impact on improving the quality of the U.S. health care system. In recent years we have seen the creation of new organizations endowed with significant funds, largely from the conversion to for-profit status of nonprofit health care plans. At the time of conversion, these plans are required to establish nonprofit foundations for the benefit of the community. In the last decade we have seen the conversion of such organizations as Blue Cross of California, which spawned two significant foundations (the California Health Care Foundation and the California Endowment), Health Net (which spawned the California Wellness Foundation), and others of less significant scale across the country.

These organizations are tripping over each other in their efforts to analyze the problems of health care access, cost, and quality, but none of them have sufficient scale to make a difference in service delivery through philanthropy alone. A strategy foundations can use for leverage is to make the public and the media aware of health policy by developing new research, disseminating information, and actively engaging the media in coverage of health care policy issues. Part of the problem here is that we actually do know that there are uninsured people, yet as a nation we simply don't care. We do know that we are far from healthy and that we shouldn't overindulge, but we choose not to do anything about it; total food consumption is on the rise, and we are as a nation getting chunkier. We do know that there is a great benefit to exercise and to wellness and health promotion, but we elect to have a different lifestyle. We know that safe sex will slow the spread of AIDs, but population groups choose not to heed the information.

Despite a recalcitrant public, foundations have had a significant impact on many of these issues through education and raising public awareness. But the issue of universal coverage may be too large for foundations to tackle in any significant way, unless they find a specific angle. They can point to the problem, dissect the issue, and galvanize government or private actors to make changes; but they can't provide enough philanthropy to cover people.

Foundations are also legally hamstrung on political advocacy with regard to expanded government coverage. The Robert Wood Johnson Foundation pushed the envelope in the 1994 elections because of their stance of apparently supporting the direction of the Clinton health policy by disseminating information about the proposals. Similarly, the Henry J. Kaiser Family Foundation continues to walk a tight line, potentially stepping over toward partisan advocacy for government reform and only through astute leadership managing to avoid crossing into overt advocacy. Judicious appointment of board members from both sides of the political aisle allows the foundation to be legitimately portrayed as unbiased. But the Kaiser Family Foundation is a good example of a foundation focused on government as a target for foundation leverage.

Much of the foundation sector's work really points to problems that can be solved only by government, but many foundations see the law that prohibits tax-exempt foundations from lobbying as not allowing them to really advocate for radical change in government policies.

So there is a search for leverage in the foundation community. For example, the Robert Wood Johnson Foundation believes it can make a big difference by focusing on substance abuse and tobacco. Similarly, the California Wellness Foundation programs on violence and violence prevention and on the role of work in health have been significant innovations and sources of leverage.

But there is much more to be done, and foundations have key opportunities to reenergize the whole of health care. They can help fill the coming leadership void by identifying and nurturing a new generation of leaders. They can support health policy research to develop new theory for health care. They can support and encourage new leadership models and new leadership practices.

Foundations need to do the following:

- Identify key leverage points at which their limited resources can be applied to greatest effect
- Coordinate among themselves so that they don't waste their resources competing with one another
- Use their power and leverage with government, the media, and policy elites to promote a more ambitious agenda for health, not simply tweak the existing health care system

Shared Leadership Challenges

It is clear that there is a leadership crisis in health care. The crisis extends from the level of values and ethics to the politics and practices of individual institutions. This critique is not intended to blame the current leaders in health care. However, the changes in health care that we examine throughout this book make the leadership challenges increasingly difficult and require us to redouble our efforts to build leadership capacities for the future.

The challenges as we enter the new millennium will be more daunting than those we have faced in the past. Therefore, this book is not meant as a personal criticism of the leadership inadequacies of those who currently lead. Rather it is a call to action for everyone in health care to recognize a recommitment to leadership and to the "leadership engine" of health care—that is, the capacity of health care organizations to encourage and develop a new generation of leaders—if we are going to be successful in the future. Noel Tichy's book *The Leadership Engine* chronicles how

General Electric (GE) develops leaders. According to Tichy, GE has ten world-class internal candidates for CEO Jack Welch's position, thanks to its leadership engine. Very few health care organizations across the country can really say they have or are generating ten world-class candidates for replacement of their current leaders.

One source of this leadership problem is the insularity in health care. There are very few leaders of large health care organizations who come from outside the health care industry. The examples tend to be extremely isolated: Russ Tobias, a former AT&T'er who ran Eli Lilly until the late 1990s, is perhaps a singular example on the pharmaceutical side; in managed care, hospitals, and health care services, leaders are, almost to a person, lifers in health care.

Health care is a unique industry in many ways, and there are all kinds of reasons why health care organizations should not be led the same way as automotive or telecommunications businesses. But the industry's unique characteristics—for example, highly professionalized employees; asymmetry of information, and other sources of market failure; the existence of third-party coverage; and the complexity of missions for nonprofit health care organizations—do not excuse health care leadership. We have a series of tired and battle-weary elites in health care, and the young Turks from the sixties are rapidly becoming the old guard. There is a deep need for new leadership and new leadership capacities in the health care industry. We need to develop leaders who know how to manage in times of change, who can stimulate organizations to innovate, and who know how to build consensus across the value landscape.

Reasons for Optimism

Although there are many leadership challenges on the horizon, there are also reasons for optimism. Organizations such as the Health Forum have committed to supporting leadership development across what CEO Kathryn Johnson calls "the 360 of health care." These efforts are to be applauded.

There are also a number of positive signs in the field. First, there is a network of thriving community-based organizations that are focused on stimulating the creation of healthier communities.

Both the Health Forum and the Health Research and Education Trust have provided leadership in fostering such networks. Local community leadership is a necessary but insufficient factor in creating a better future.

The second key area for optimism is the recent political energy around meaningful reform of Medicare. Properly designed, a healthy Medicare program could be a platform for universal coverage. Remember, there is no such thing as voluntary universal coverage. Universality requires action by the federal government. Although state experimentation is valuable in developing and testing possible health policy alternatives, it is inconceivable that states will spontaneously reach universal coverage on their own.

Unless the federal government mandates universal coverage, we are likely to go through another thousand years of worrying about the problem of the uninsured. Imagine a political compromise at the federal level, one that coalesces around the concepts and values of floors and ceilings, guaranteeing a basic floor for all Americans and equally the right to trade up with one's own money to a ceiling of one's choice.

Another element of a compromise would be to require individuals to purchase insurance, instead of requiring employers to provide it. The tax system could be changed so as to create an inducement; the tax benefit employers currently receive would need to be put in the hands of individuals. Simply mandating that individuals purchase insurance is not enough. Clearly, there would have to be a tax-based subsidy for the poor and the working poor. The political compromise would then revolve around the degree to which the contribution toward this mandate would be in the form of a premium, which would be a regressive form of tax, or in the form of a payroll tax, which would clearly be more of a progressive form of payment. In simplistic form, an individual mandate could have appeal for Republicans—as individuals taking responsibility—but it would be a universal mandate with appeal for the Democrats.

Medicare reform could be the central policy instrument of the future. One of the reasons the Clinton plan failed was that nobody had ever actually seen a health insurance purchasing cooperative (HIPC). Few had experienced managed competition as a model (except for those at CalPers or Stanford University). Suppose we were to make Medicare+Choice work as a public policy. Medicare+Choice allows Medicare recipients to select among competing health plans of all types. Imagine that 30 or 40 percent of our elderly population were in a managed care framework and were content with their plan. Why wouldn't such a program available to all the public be a solution for the future?

This is but one vision. We will explore this and others in the chapters that follow. But meaningful change in health care will not come about from ideas, scenarios, or policy alternatives alone. It will require leadership at all levels of the health care system.

Chapter Three

New Millennium Drivers of Change

As we move into the new millennium, a series of important driving forces will eventually culminate in massive transformation of the American health care system, as described throughout this book. Many of these forces have been building for a long time, and some are the result of more recent changes, but in combination they will drive our future.

The Coming Public Discontent

As we look out to the near term, we are very likely to see a reemergence of the kind of public dissatisfaction with health care we saw in 1994, which led to health care reform. Louis Harris and Associates has conducted public opinion surveys on satisfaction with health care over the past twenty years. The results indicate that by 1997–98, discontent with health care among the U.S. public was beginning to rise to 1994 levels. Public dissatisfaction has risen because health benefits have eroded, consumers have had to pay more for health care, and the negative dimensions of managed care are becoming more apparent. Dissatisfaction with health care is highest among the rising number of uninsured, and among a large proportion (over a quarter) of the public that experiences being uninsured in any two-year period. In addition to dissatisfaction, anxiety also is high among this marginally insured group.

What is remarkable about this public discontent is that it has been rising in the last few years despite sustained economic prosperity. Normally one would expect discontent to be parallel with economic circumstances, and indeed the long-term satisfaction has shifted with the economic times: satisfaction tends to be higher in times of economic prosperity. But in this period of economic expansion, we have seen a break from the historical pattern: there is economic prosperity superimposed on a structural long-term trend toward discontent and dissatisfaction with the health care system. If we were to dip into recession or a period of economic slowdown, public discontent would intensify; because employee benefits and the welfare system were cut at the height of the economic expansion, the vulnerability of health insurance coverage would become very apparent to those who are marginally employed when and if a recession hits.

Reluctantly Empowered Consumers

There is increased consumerization in health care, but much of the rhetoric of consumerization is overblown. The prevailing theory of health care consumerism is that consumers will gleefully trade up to more expensive forms of care with their own money and that the consumer trends in the marketplace are well developed (much in the way that other markets for services and consumer goods are well developed, with defined segments and well-established patterns of behavior).

The reason it is premature to take this kind of consumerist view is that historically health care has not been a consumer good. Most consumers have not had to pay a higher share of their health care costs out of pocket over the last thirty years. Third-party insurance coverage has paid for a rising share of total health care costs until recently. It is only in the last two to three years that we've seen signs of reversal: the rate of increase in expenditures by consumers is now greater than the rate of increase in health expenditures as a whole. This change suggests that out-of-pocket spending, the use of discretionary income, and discretionary choices in health care will become more of a factor. One thing we know from twenty years of public opinion research in health care is that when consumers pay more out of pocket for health care, they get very, very cranky.

Consumers are starting to pay more out of pocket for health care, but they are also becoming more active consumers. There are eight key factors underlying the increased degree of consumerization in health care.

1. *Education.* The baby boom generation and the cohorts that follow it have higher rates of college education than previous cohorts had. A key insight is that people who have attended at least one year of college behave in much the same way as those who have attended for four years; so a youth population in which 60 to 70 percent receive some amount of college education is a precursor of a more sophisticated, skeptical, and demanding middle-class public. Education, then, is a primary driver behind consumerization in health.

2. *The shift from defined benefit to defined contribution.* The second key driver behind consumerization in health care is the behavior of large employers and public sector programs such as Medicare and Medicaid. Both the large employers and Medicare and Medicaid are moving toward managed care models in which there is both a greater choice of plans made available to the enrollees and a concomitant shift away from a defined-benefit model to a defined-contribution model. This shift is analogous to what happened to pension plans in the 1980s. Up until that time, those who were fortunate enough to have pension plans were covered on a defined-benefit basis; that is, the pension benefits were prescribed in advance. The shift to defined contribution basically put employees in the position of making their own investments in a 401(k) or other kind of plan to provide for their retirement. The model in health care is patterned somewhat after the pension plan model; primarily, however, the health care model is related to the notion of managed competition, a system in which consumers trade up with their own money to a higher level of coverage, superior benefits, or perceived improvements in quality or customer service.

3. *Relentless media coverage.* The third factor that is driving consumerization is relentless coverage of health care in the media. This has made consumers more informed and more skeptical. Simultaneously it has led to increased consumerization in the health care field as more and more articles are written and more and more television programs are dedicated to the consumer side of health care and to helping consumers understand their rights in navigating through the system. The coverage comes through the

mainstream media, in both print and electronic form, but also increasingly in much more sophisticated forms: targeted newsletters, community interest groups, and electronic communities.

4. *Cyberchondria.* The fourth driver is a special form of electronic community: that of cyberchondriacs, people who use the Internet to seek health care information. This term was coined by a Harvard graduate student and brought into popular usage by Humphrey Taylor, chairman of Louis Harris and Associates. According to Harris, sixty million people searched the World Wide Web for health care information in 1998; Harris estimates that this number will rise to seventy million in 1999. The growth of the Internet—arguably the fastest-growing new technology in history—has generated explosive growth in the number of people who search the Web for health care information related to specific diseases.

In the Harris poll, 68 percent of the people on-line say they used the Web in the previous twelve months to look for "health care information related to any particular disease or medical condition." Other Harris data show that the on-line population (from home, office, school, or elsewhere) has risen to 44 percent of adults (that is, eighty-eight million people). The cyberchondriacs using the Web to search for health care information therefore account for 68 percent of that on-line population, or sixty million adults, a staggering number. The Harris survey also shows that the value and success of the Web is remarkable; nine out of every ten (91 percent) of these people say that the last time they searched the Web for health care information, they found what they wanted.

The diseases that generate the greatest use of the Web are depression (19 percent of cyberchondriacs), allergies or sinus problems (16 percent), cancer (15 percent), bipolar disorder (14 percent), arthritis or rheumatism (10 percent), high blood pressure (10 percent), migraine (9 percent), anxiety disorder (9 percent), heart disease (8 percent), and sleep disorders (8 percent). Many Web sites contain multiple linkages, but the sites people believe they referenced most often were those of medical societies (40 percent), patient advocacy groups or support groups (32 percent), pharmaceutical companies (20 percent), and hospitals (16 percent). As the Internet continues to grow, we are all likely to become cyberchondriacs to some degree, forever changing the way we access medical care.

5. *Direct-to-consumer (DTC) advertising.* To some degree, the consumerization of health care is driven not only by demand pull, as it were, but also by supply push—in other words, the marketing behavior of both health plans and pharmaceuticals. Health plans, such as Oxford Health Plans and United HealthCare, have tried to position themselves as consumer-friendly and consumer-responsive (although HMOs find it very difficult to differentiate themselves in terms of their customer service). Perhaps the best sustained example to date has been Blue Shield of California, with its Access Plus HMO, which includes self-referring to specialists, and, in late 1998, its release of its www.mylifepath.com Web site, which provides consumers with information across the continuum of health care. Blue Shield's strategy is discussed in more detail in Chapter Nine.

In the pharmaceutical area, DTC advertising has been increasing in the late 1990s at a rate of around 30 percent compounded annually. Once prevented by regulation from advertising aggressively, pharmaceutical companies now see DTC advertising as a major source of stimulating demand for their product; they spent $1.3 billion on DTC advertising in 1998 alone. This has had two key effects: (1) it has built brand awareness and product awareness in the minds of end users (consumers), who are increasingly taking medications for chronic conditions in increasingly crowded and competitive therapeutic categories—cholesterol management, cardiovascular diseases, asthma, allergy, and other forms of respiratory ailments; and (2) more directly, it has encouraged users to visit their doctors and ask for the product by name.

DTC advertising is being used somewhat as a blunt instrument, however. The pharmaceutical industry has gone overboard on this strategy. There is the potential for DTC advertising to backfire on the pharmaceutical industry in the long run, because the strategy is alienating the managed care health plans; and it won't be long before that discontent is felt by consumers and government as they come to realize that the rising price and utilization of these drugs are partly a result of DTC advertising. Nevertheless, DTC advertising has been a major and significant contributor to consumerization in the later part of the 1990s.

6. *Advocacy groups.* Patient advocacy groups and disease advocacy groups are also drivers of consumerization. This phenomenon

gained momentum with the AIDS epidemic and the rise of AIDS advocacy groups. Over the last decade and a half, we have seen a wide range of disease-related advocacy groups develop very aggressive approaches toward legislators and providers of services to ensure they are responsive to each particular group's needs for treatment and research. These advocacy groups have increasing power in the health system and have demonstrated an ability to significantly change the course of public policy—for example, changing the regulations for breast cancer treatment coverage so that insurers cover various forms of breast reconstruction following surgery. Advocacy groups are likely to grow in importance in the future, and the Internet has provided a platform and vehicle for creating and sustaining them.

7. *Self-care.* Increases in self-diagnosis and self-medication, including the use of self-testing equipment (which has become much more prevalent in the last decade), have driven the consumerization of health care. This is part of a broader trend of consumers taking charge of their own health and health care. Self-medication and the use of a whole host of vitamins and other forms of supplement have led to an enormous growth in the dietary, supplement, and vitamin industry. For example, according to the November 23, 1998, issue of *Time* magazine, there are 7.5 million users of St. John's wort, a plant extract with antidepressant properties; 7.3 million users of echinacea, which is taken to prevent colds and flu; and 10.8 million users of gingko biloba, which is taken for all kinds of ailments. Consumers spent more than $12 billion on natural supplements in 1998, and sales continue to grow at 10 percent per year.

8. *Complementary and alternative medicine.* Related to the rise in self-diagnosis and self-medication is the rise of alternative medicine. According to the same *Time* article, consumers spent some $28 billion on alternative health care in 1998. Alternative medicine is on the rise for several reasons: consumer preferences for natural products; increasing diversity in the population and influence of other cultures from around the world, bringing not only folk remedies but also different cultural responses to disease; the rise in spiritualism and New Age concepts of well-being; recognition of a broader definition of health; and increased skepticism on the part of a sophisticated public that conventional medical techniques are the only solutions to people's health problems.

In no small way is the rise of alternative medicine also attributed to patients' satisfaction with the results of some of these forms of therapy. Chiropractors have loyal followings of patients who feel that their backs got better. Patients who have quit smoking or have seen significant relief in their arthritis or dermatological conditions through acupuncture swear by that remedy. The conventional medical establishment has been forced—rather reluctantly—to embrace many of these therapies. There is evidence everywhere of the mainstreaming of alternative therapies, not the least of which is in managed care organizations like Kaiser, which has created significant programs incorporating alternative therapy.

It is also likely that alternative therapy will receive more legitimacy through the research process as university-based programs start receiving significant funding from foundations interested in the field of alternative therapy. For example, the Bernard Osher Foundation in San Francisco gave $10 million to the University of California–San Francisco (UCSF) to establish the Osher Center for Integrative Medicine. According to a UCSF press release, "The center's mission is to search for the most effective treatments by combining non-traditional and traditional approaches that address all aspects of health and wellness—biological, psychological, social, and spiritual." New research by prestigious academic medical centers is likely to add legitimacy to the wave of consumer interest in alternative and complementary therapies.

The Rubble of the Managed Care Revolution

Managed care has significantly altered the landscape of American health care. Managed care is certainly in some disarray as we close the millennium. Many ask what will come next. Although managed care has to evolve, it would be wrong to assume that managed care is going to disappear. There are few other viable alternatives if we are going to contain costs and improve quality.

The notion that the field can be left to consumers engaging providers through their medical savings account is not only naive but clearly an ideological nirvana that is unlikely to happen. There have to be mediating organizations, and in most other countries, government plays a significant role in that mediation. In the United States it is much more likely that we will have a mixed public-private form of intermediary between patients and providers.

This is not because there needs to be interference in the doctor-patient relationship but because making health care available only to those individuals who are able to pay for it is neither possible nor desirable if we are going to preserve social order. There will have to be insurance, and there will have to be some form of sub-sidy for both the poor and the elderly to ensure adequate access to some form of health care.

So managed care is not going away, nor is third-party coverage. But managed care needs to transform itself, and at this point the industry is caught in a dilemma: the need for innovation comes at a time when the resources available to managed care have been severely constrained. As we have seen, the profitability of managed care companies has been significantly eroded through the 1990s, and these companies' ability to revive Wall Street's interest in their longer-term future has been constrained to some degree. We will explore the strategic alternatives for managed care health plans in Chapter Nine. The current trend is for plans to be either virtual single payers or large-scale vertically integrated HMOs, but neither model has been perfect.

The Fruits of Innovation

New clinical and biotechnology innovations will emerge because of the enormous investment made by the pharmaceutical industry in R&D and because of the increasing investment in basic bio-medical research through the National Institutes of Health. The rise of the new biology and the streamlining of FDA approvals have brought a flood of new products to market in the late 1990s. For example, the mean FDA approval time for new molecular entities (NMEs) in 1987 was 32.4 months. By 1997 that figure had dropped exactly in half to 16.2 months, largely as a result of the reforms in 1994, whereby the pharmaceutical industry was required to pay a fee to ensure the smoother operation of FDA approvals. Over the same period, the number of approvals almost doubled. In 1987, twenty NMEs were approved. By 1997, that figure had jumped to thirty-nine—almost exactly double. Indeed, the average of 1996 and 1997 was more than twice the 1987 level.

The pharmaceutical industry not only created a range of new products but also has indulged itself in what one might call venture-capital pricing—that is, pricing the product to capture all the lifetime profit for the product in its first two or three years on the market. Companies are using this approach partly to recoup the costs of R&D (which are estimated by the industry to exceed $400 million for any individual drug) and to compensate for the fact that the moment in the sun that a new blockbuster drug might enjoy has become shorter and shorter. Tagamet, the first h-2 antagonist medication for stomach ulcers, had almost a decade-long run; Xantac, the next big player, had somewhat close to half that time because of competing blockbuster therapies. Now blockbusters enjoy one to two years of enormous profit before an even better mousetrap comes along. But aside from these rationales, the industry has also simply priced new products as the market will bear; and given the monopoly status of these products, the market bears a very high price.

Pharmaceutical companies have overcome the obstacles of managed care. As we discussed in Chapter One, they have sophisticated pharmaco-economic teams to negotiate the presence of their products on the formulary, and they have understood how to use both legislative action and sophisticated marketing to ensure that their products are not cut out of either Medicaid or private sector formularies. They have been significantly investing in DTC advertising as well as expanding their sales forces for detailing physicians. This is the business model for the pharmaceutical industry in the late 1990s, and industry leaders anticipate that these good times will continue rolling into the future.

The innovative power of the contemporary pharmaceutical and medical technology industry has significant long-term implications for the health services industry. In a recent ten-year forecast produced for the Robert Wood Johnson Foundation (available from the foundation), the Institute for the Future (IFTF) cited eight interesting areas of new technology that were likely to emerge. These technology areas were identified based on IFTF interviews with leading experts as part of their overall forecast for health care.

1. *Rational drug design:* the use of computers to design drugs that target a particular receptor.
2. *Advances in imaging:* the use of new imaging technologies, such as electron-beam CT harmonic ultrasound, high-resolution

PET, and functional MRI, to look at the form and function of organs that were once examined only in surgery.

3. *Minimally invasive surgery:* the use of miniaturized devices, digitized imaging, and vascular catheters in neurosurgery, cardiology, and interventional radiology.

4. *Genetic mapping and testing:* the identification and testing of genes and genetic interactions that cause disease.

5. *Gene therapy:* the use of site-specific genes to treat a variety of inherited or acquired diseases.

6. *Vaccines:* the use of vaccines to bolster immune systems, to target tumors, or to immunize against viruses. Delivery methods including oral and nasal sprays will simplify the vaccination process.

7. *Artificial blood:* the use of recombinant hemoglobin using *e. coli* to create a blood substitute.

8. *Xenotransplantation:* the transplantation of tissues and organs (primarily bone marrow and solid organs) from animals into humans.

These and other technologies will open up exciting new methods of diagnosis, treatment, and even cure for a wide range of diseases, such as cancer, diabetes, and heart disease; but they also are likely to have a profound impact on the health care system by increasing the costs of care and challenging an overstretched managed care industry.

The Promise of the Web but Lack of Information Technology Infrastructure

The Internet is transforming every industry it touches, and it is likely that health care will be no exception. For example, health-related portals are emerging, such as Web MD, a recent start-up with heavy corporate backing from life sciences giant Dupont. Web MD aims to own the point of interaction between physicians and the Internet, to allow physicians to do research on-line and to serve their patients. Web MD is merging with Healtheon, another high-flying, well-funded Internet company founded by Silicon Valley legend Jim Clark (founder of both Silicon Graphics and Netscape). Healtheon has its sights set on resolving the administrative inefficiencies in the back office of health care. Channelpoint is another start-up with impressive backing; it is intent on revolutionizing the way health plans reach small businesses and individual consumers—currently a horrendously inefficient process that absorbs 10 percent of the health care premium for small-group insurance.

These companies, and a host of others, have impressive venture backers, sophisticated corporate partners, and a compelling vision. But they will be fighting an uphill battle. Health care is a knowledge- and information-intensive industry, yet it has not demonstrated an overarching commitment to the standardized use of new information tools and technologies. This lack of commitment is in sharp contrast to the behavior of other service industries. Overcoming this resistance will be a significant factor in the future transformation of health care. Again, the IFTF's recent report points to some of the major trends in information technology.

• *Automation of basic business processes.* The transaction standards mandated in 1996 by the Health Insurance Portability and Accountability Act will move plans and providers early in the next decade toward automation of claims, submission, adjudication, patient eligibility, coordination of benefits, and referral authorizations, fueling the growth of Internet and non-Internet-enabled solutions. In addition, other clinical administrative processes, such as patient scheduling, test ordering, and results reporting, will continue to penetrate the outpatient setting.

• *Clinical information interfaces.* An electronic medical record has proven to be a very difficult technology to bring to bear on medical care, even though many of the basic building blocks have been put in place. Over the next decade, the availability of computers, sophisticated decision-support systems, and voice recognition will create interfaces that are more clinician-friendly. Lower-priced equipment; younger, computer-savvy clinicians; and the move of physicians into larger groups will together cause a slow but real diffusion of computerized medical records in the years after 2005.

• *Data analysis.* In the next few years, administrative and claims data sets will be extensively mined by clinicians, researchers, and managed care organizations alike. This will lead to better understanding of a population's future health status and improved ability to risk-adjust payments to health plans and providers.

- *Telehealth.* A combination of computer-supported case management, remote telemetry via sensors, and better-informed patients will create new ways of delivering health care. The vast increase in health information available via the Internet and through a whole series of potentially linked devices could have profound effects on the health system of the future.

Rediscovery of Community

Even though much of health care financing and policy direction comes from the national level, health care is nevertheless a local good. Therefore, leadership at the local community level can make an enormous difference in improving the health and health care of the public. There is a move in U.S. health care that could be termed the *rediscovery of community* as people become increasingly interested in understanding the role communities play in fostering health. The Healthier Communities movement and the Healthy Cities movement have been embraced by a number of different organizations, the Health Forum and the Health Research and Education Trust being perhaps the two most notable examples. It is interesting that both organizations are now aligned under the American Hospital Association umbrella. Both of these organizations have played important roles in fostering an interest in thinking about healthier communities and in providing a series of ongoing educational and learning collaboratives whereby communities could truly develop a broader perspective of health. For example, South Bend, Indiana, under the leadership of local health care leaders Phil Newbold and Carl Ellison, has gone a long way in its community to integrate the concept of health into its school system, its business community, and its civic governments.

Understanding the importance of community in the healing process is just part of the potential future impact of this rediscovery of community. At another level, community is the logical locus of rationalization of health care delivery and is perhaps the unit of analysis for meaningful change in terms of financing health care. Although it is true that federal reform would be required to ensure universal coverage, cities and metropolitan areas have an opportunity to shape the structure and organization of health care. Significant actors, such as local business coalitions, can help determine the future course of the health system within the community. This has certainly been the case in a variety of cities across the United States, including Minneapolis, the San Francisco Bay Area, Orlando, and Rochester.

The Default Future

The drivers we have examined—public discontent, consumerization, managed care, technological innovation, the promise of the Internet despite an immature information technology infrastructure, and the growth of community—will combine to affect the health system of the future. But they will not combine in a positive way without the leadership to pull these drivers together. Allowed to move on uncontrolled, these forces will drive us to a default future that is not particularly pleasant.

• *Rising uninsured.* The first element of the default future is the rising number of uninsured. By 1997, there were 43.1 million uninsured Americans. That number is 12 million higher than it would have been had the penetration of insurance in the employment sector remained at the 1987 level. In other words, a significant part of the increase in the number of uninsured has really been because of deterioration in health coverage within the business community rather than because of unemployment or underemployment in the community. A full 80 percent of the uninsured are working people and their families.

• *Massive shift from defined benefit to defined contribution.* As we have seen, both the public and private sectors are going to move increasingly from a defined-benefit model to a defined-contribution model, creating a world where consumers are going to be trading up with their own money.

• *Consumers pay more, reluctantly.* Consumers are going to pay more no matter what. Unless we radically change the course of health care, the consumer will be paying more out of pocket for their health care. This is true for both those in employment and those who are under Medicare. They will do so reluctantly.

• *Big Ugly Buyers.* Big Ugly Buyers (see Chapter Seven) will play a continued role in health care, concentrating their purchasing power up the health care food chain. The role of big purchasers in health care is not going to disappear. Potentially, they will become less interested as they shift from defined benefit to defined contribution and control their financial exposure to rising health care costs. But in the short run, the Big Ugly Buyers, Medicare and Medicaid in particular, will continue to have a very important role in the purchase of health care.

• *Managed care defanged over quality.* It is somewhat ironic that we've suckered HMOs into doing the job of cost containment, and now, having lured them into it through the promise of profits, we are going to regulate them. In the name of quality, or at least choice, we may end up preventing them from doing cost containment. The default future is one in which managed care is reluctantly hanging around health care even though managed care is not a particularly profitable or particularly effective business.

• *Health costs on the rise.* With managed care defanged, with the easy pickings of managed care taken, and with the tremendous pressures of a population that is both aging and enamored of all new technologies that come on the scene, health costs inevitably seem to be on the rise again with little prospect of meaningful control.

• *Wall Street disappointed with health services.* Wall Street is unlikely to be happy with health services if these trends continue. Wall Street may be delirious with the mainstream pharmaceutical industry and, to a lesser extent, with the biotechnology and medical devices sector, but they are bitterly disappointed in the recent performance of health care services. Indeed, ironically the most successful health-related mutual funds have been those that studiously avoided investment in health care services.

• *Pharmaceuticals on a roll—at least for a while.* As we have discussed, the pharmaceutical industry is on an enormous roll, at least for now. Increasingly over the next three to five years, however, this prosperity will be questioned by the public sector, by Medicare and Medicaid as payers, and by the private sector. It would be foolish for the pharmaceutical industry to extrapolate their current euphoric market forward into the future.

Chapter Four

The Challenges of Change

The health care system faces five important challenges as it tries to change. In some cases, these challenges are uniquely American and flow from our belief in pluralism, competition, and the market, or from the fact that we have a huge economy, are a large country, and have a diverse population. The first challenge—one not unique to the United States—is to resolve the tension between health and health care. Increasingly, the science of population health tells us that medical care is not the only factor behind improved health status. The second key challenge is to find a theoretical framework for health policy beyond managed competition—the prevailing theory over the last twenty years. The third, related challenge is to find ways to make community-based integrated health care systems work more effectively. They hold great promise but we have failed to make them a reality. The fourth challenge is to clarify the fuzzy boundaries between for-profit and nonprofit health care. Finally, the fifth challenge is regional diversity. The United States is a big country with tremendous regional variation in health care financing and delivery. It is important to address these challenges as we try to find a viable future.

Health Versus Health Care

When Americans talk about health care, they usually mean the service provided by doctors and hospitals, maybe even HMOs and pharmaceutical companies. But there is a growing realization around the world that health is determined more by life circumstances, livelihood, and lifestyle than by medical care. By various

53

estimates, only 10 to 25 percent of the improvement in health status can really be attributed to medical care interventions. The rest is the legacy of improved nutrition, improved public safety, and most important, improvements in income, education, and income distribution in society. The realization that these so-called population health factors are the crucial determinants of health requires us to broaden our definition of health and health care.

Broadly defined, health is the well-being of a population. Health indicators that one would look to as measures of success include such macrostatistics as life expectancy, morbidity, and mortality data. By that benchmark, U.S. health care is no great bargain, with excessive expenditure for inferior outcomes, at least as measured at the societal level by life expectancy and infant mortality. (See Table 4.1 for a comparison of health statistics for six countries.) True, the United States has more high technology than most countries (the number of magnetic resonance imaging [MRI] machines per million people is a plausible measure of technological sophistication), but high tech does not necessarily determine high expenditure, which depends on utilization and the prices for use of these technologies, as the Japanese experience shows. Japan has more MRI machines per million population than the United States, but much lower costs. The United States does provide a lot of medical care, and most of it is very high quality, but as we will discuss further, medical care alone does not create health.

In 1996, the *British Medical Journal* published two important papers, one comparing life expectancy increases among all the developed countries, the other comparing increases in life expectancy among the fifty states of the United States. The results in the two studies were remarkably similar: both indicated that the single most important explanatory variable in improvement in life expectancy was the income distribution in the society. In other words, those countries with a tight income distribution (that is, not much disparity between the income circumstances of rich and poor), such as Japan, were experiencing rapid increases in life expectancy compared to countries with a wider discrepancy between rich and poor. Similarly, the U.S. study showed that those states with a larger income disparity had a lower rate of increase of life expectancy than did the states with a tighter income distribution, such as Wisconsin or Minnesota.

Table 4.1. International Health Comparisons.

Country	HC/GDP (percent)	Population over 65 (percent)	MRI per million	Female Life Expectancy (years)	Infant Mortality (per 000)
United States	14.2	12.2	15.5	79.2	9.2
Germany	10.5	15.3	4.8	79.5	7.1
France	9.6	15.4	2.1	81.9	5.0
Canada	9.2	12.1	1.3	81.3	6.0
Japan	7.2	14.7	20.1	82.8	4.6
United Kingdom	6.9	15.8	3.4	79.7	7.9

Source: Organization for Economic Co-operation and Development (OECD), 1998.

At a cursory glance, the policy prescription might be to redistribute income more aggressively. However, income redistribution is not a core value in the United States, so it is unlikely that we will ever see massive income redistribution on the socialized model of Sweden or Japan. In fact, trends toward individualism, privatization, and pluralism, even in the more socialized and democratized countries, suggest that massive income distribution is not necessarily the direction of the contemporary political economy in advanced countries. Indeed, many countries that have had well-established welfare states (for example, Sweden and the United Kingdom) are seeing a greater role for the private sector in many areas, such as telecommunications and transportation, and even in the organization and management of their social welfare system.

It is important to recognize that access to medical care does play a key role in improving health status. The literature and research over the years has indicated that those without access to routine health care suffer from health problems and health status issues that can be directly attributable to their lack of medical care. But it is also true that in taking an overall view, the most salient gains in health status can be achieved through broader social and economic interventions. For example, there is growing understanding of the degree to which work and the organizational structure contribute to stress on the individual and lack of health improvement, or health gain, as it is termed in the United Kingdom.

A recent report by the Institute for the Future noted the following: "Whether social class is measured by income, education, employment grade, or prestige, it determines the resources that are available to meet life's challenges and therefore influences the control one has in shaping life. The 1980 publication of the Black Report showed the statistical association between illness and social class in England and Wales. Physical and mental health, the statistics showed, ran parallel to social rank. With the introduction of universal health care through the National Health Service, these differences in health status among different socioeconomic groups actually became greater!"

Thus, even in a country with universal health care coverage and a highly socialized and supposedly equitable approach to the delivery of health services, there were marked death rate differences among the strata of British society. This indicates that the drivers of health status and disease burden have much to do with the relative stress and other factors associated with socioeconomic status in general and with conditions in the workplace in particular.

Differentiating between health and health care and understanding the role of each are important challenges our society must face if our health system is to move forward. The focus on determinants of health is manifested in a number of different ways. It is evident in the interest shown by the leading health care foundations, such as the Robert Wood Johnson Foundation, and other organizations, such as the AHA, the Health Forum, the Public Health Leadership Institute, and the Health Research and Education Trust, in promoting a broader definition of health and in focusing on the determinants of community health as goals for health care systems.

The AHA, in particular, has adopted a mission and vision of "healthier communities and community networks of care." The goals of the AHA are increasingly focused on improving the broader health of the community, although their constituents are heavily focused on providing health services and are keenly interested in continued financial sustenance for those health services.

As we discussed in Chapter Two, this creates tension for the hospital sector if, as the population health literature indicates, the factors that really improve health status have a lot more to do with income distribution than with medical care. Hospitals have very little opportunity to affect those key determinants of health. Ironically, from an extreme population health perspective, the best thing that hospitals can do to improve health is to employ people. Nevertheless, the focus on health as a fundamental vision for a hospital association must be applauded.

Second, the tension between health and health care is being played out in the recent strategic redirection of the Robert Wood Johnson Foundation, the nation's leading private philanthropic organization focused on health. Recognizing the distinction and tension between health and health care, the foundation has gone so far as to divide its grant-giving activities into two program areas: one focused on health and one focused on health care. One could argue that when the leading grant maker in the field divides its focus, it is driving a wedge between health and health care; but the foundation's commitment to a separate and distinct focus on health does help reinforce a key need in the marketplace for better understanding among physicians, the public, and policymakers that if our society is to achieve meaningful improvement in health status, we must give much greater attention to the fundamental drivers and determinants of health, not simply to improvements in the quality and accessibility of medical care.

At a conference in 1999, Steven Schroeder, president and CEO of the Robert Wood Johnson Foundation, pointed to the significant health status gains that have been achieved in this country through attention to the determinants of health. He cites as examples the enormous backlash against the tobacco industry even by Republican leaders, who had been long-term industry supporters and defenders. In recent years, Republicans have moved to a much more neutral, if not absolutely confrontational, position against the tobacco lobbies. Schroeder also points to other significant improvements over the last twenty years, including increase in the use of seat belts and other forms of public safety, reduction in murder rates across the country, and decreased use of drugs in the community. Despite the media's increasing attention to drugs and crime in local and national news, the long-run trend for violent crime, drug use, and tobacco is down. However, critics legitimately can still point to the alarming upturn in consumption of marijuana, cigarettes, and other drugs in certain younger populations. It is interesting to note that we are more drug and crime obsessed while simultaneously we are more drug and crime free. We are more fitness and nutritionally conscious, just as we as a nation get more obese and more sedentary. The popular culture is at odds with the facts.

If the positive future of health is to be realized in the United States, greater attention has to be paid, in the media and in all levels of decision making, to the determinants of health. There are a number of organizations advocating such points of view, but it is difficult to get the public's attention on these issues. The public likes wellness and prevention and health promotion as general concepts. But when it comes to the practical realization that redistribution of income or education are more effective mechanisms for improving health status than is cardiac surgery or even jogging, the whole thing really smacks too much of socialism for the average American.

So here rests the irony in the health versus health care debate. The things that work to improve health status are politically unacceptable to a population that believes in individualism and that equates health care with access to esoteric medical services and not with the social and economic infrastructure that creates health. Selling a focus on the determinants of health is a difficult challenge for all the elites who favor a more health-oriented position, and it is certainly a source of tension within the health care provider community.

Finding a Framework Beyond Managed Competition

The second key challenge of change is to overcome the vacuum of theory in which the United States finds itself in the late 1990s. Nor are we alone: around the world, managed competition was embraced as a possible future framework for health and health services. As we discussed in Chapter One, Alain Enthoven and Paul Ellwood created a vision of managed competition in which vertically integrated health plans competed head-to-head, on the basis of price and quality, for informed consumers. These consumers were to select among the competing health plans when they were well and live with the consequences of these choices when they were sick. The idea was that consumers would make much more cost-conscious decisions about their choice of health plan because they were making decisions with their own money when they were well and presumably rational. (This certainly makes more sense than the market alternatives proposed by some who suggest that health care is like any other good or service. It's tough to be cost-conscious when one is under anesthetic—the situation in which most health costs are incurred.)

The notion is that this mixed marvel of competition and control would provide incentives to integrated health systems to be both more efficient and high quality. Managed competition would also provide an incentive to cost-conscious consumers to be careful and prudent in their selection of health plans. And perhaps most important, the fact that health plans and integrated systems would be caring for a defined population gave them an incentive to care about the health of the population and about the determinants of health. Thus market forces, large-scale organization, and population health were brought together in an alignment of incentives for one wonderful moment when health care all made sense. Everyone could give the keynote address; it was like a rap song: "Capitate, integrate, communicate, yo bro'—I wanna be an HMO."

The managed competition model had great appeal as a theoretical construct throughout the 1980s and early 1990s, and it was really the intellectual framework behind the rise of managed care in both the public and private sector, and was the major stimulus for the creation of integrated health systems.

Making Community-Based Integrated Systems Work

There was considerable euphoria in the late 1980s and early 1990s around the concept of integration. It was argued that if health systems could vertically integrate in local communities, they would be better able to improve the health of those communities and provide greater continuity across the continuum of care and more improved efficiencies in terms of the distribution of services. In effect, the goal was to try to emulate Kaiser and the staff-model

HMOs, which ironically had actually stopped growing around 1990, just about the time the integrated health care mantra began.

The trend toward integrated systems was amplified by think tanks and consultants who argued that health care reform would lead to a massive and rapid shift to capitation—"The Russians are coming! The Russians are coming!" Panicked, hospital CEOs bought physicians' practices (particularly primary care), and some even got into the HMO business.

Then such analysts as Jeff Goldsmith questioned the validity of actual integration, pointing to the fact that true integration in other industries never really yields much of an economic payoff either for the corporation or its consumers. James Robinson, the Berkeley health economist, has argued more recently from a theoretical perspective that vertical integration rarely makes sense. Overall, *virtual* integration—that is, smooth linkages between vendors, suppliers, and distributors, mediated through contracts and technology—is a much, much more effective mechanism for providing flexibility, efficiency, effectiveness, and consumer satisfaction. For example, many industries, from automobiles to food to clothing, are linked through virtual supply and distribution chains rather than through tight ownership relationships; and certainly the Internet is the mother of all examples of virtual integration.

Virtual integration became a lightning rod for experimentation by health systems and by managed care organizations through the 1990s. Many of the managed care plans (such as HealthNet and PacifiCare in California) emphasized network models in which they delegated care to capitated medical groups. Other HMOs, such as United HealthCare, Aetna U.S. Healthcare, and Cigna Healthplans, grew through the development of more diverse relationships with individual physicians and independent practice associations. Similarly, hospitals created virtual relationships (in the form of partnerships and joint ventures with their physicians). However, virtual integration, as it has played out so far, seems to work well only as long as you have virtual illnesses. The lack of information infrastructure, the pluralism and fragmentation of the health care system, and the overarching problems of coordination of care across all the various aspects of health services really have made virtual integration more of a conceptual triumph than an actual triumph on the ground.

In early 1999 a CEO of a South Florida health system remarked to me, "We did all those California things: we bought physician practices, we started an HMO joint venture with a commercial insurer, and we have a PHO that we folded all our doctors into. We are losing money on all of that stuff. The gatekeeper model is dying, it's all open access, and we don't know how to run physician practices anyway. Nobody does. We make money in our little hospitals where we are the sole community provider."

In most communities, health systems are not yet providing the kind of coordinated service that integration once promised, be it virtual or actual. Part of the problem here is that community-based integration requires the coordination of various actors in a trusted environment. And indeed if one goes back to the thesis of managed competition, it is predicated on exclusive, trusting relationships among the hospitals, the health plans, and the physicians in these integrated systems. However, this reality never materialized, and community-based integrated systems rarely, if ever, involved exclusive, trusting relationships between plan and hospital and physician.

Even in the most advanced managed care markets, such as San Diego, Minneapolis, and Portland, physician groups tended to affiliate with many competing systems, and exclusive relationships were rare. Indeed San Diego, which is perhaps the most advanced managed care market and where exclusivity of vertical integration went the furthest, has probably fared the worst in terms of local institutions flourishing, because of the brutal competition on which these systems embarked. For example, the annual conference sponsored by the University of California–San Diego, which focused on trends in the San Diego managed care marketplace, used to draw a wide national audience in 1993 and 1994, when managed competition was on a roll as the theory du jour, and integrated systems were the future. The conference was attended by a range of people from around the country eager to understand how to become like San Diego. By 1998, virtually all attendees were from San Diego County, and there was little or no interest by anyone outside San Diego in the travails of the San Diego health care system. This is testimony to the turnaround in thinking about the future that has occurred in the 1990s.

The seeming abandonment of community-based integrated systems as the clarion cry for health care is troubling because the concept of an integrated health system focused on serving a local community was not wrong in its intent. Perhaps we failed in execution. Perhaps we lost commitment. But the situation seems to illustrate the American problem in health policy, namely that we like to move swiftly from one bad idea to another bad idea, or even from one good idea to another good idea, without fully implementing any of the ideas in the process. Fads and fashions come and go, and no one really makes full-time and long-term commitment to implementing any of these ideas. Uwe Reinhardt, a health economist at Princeton, has called this "management by Modern Healthcare," named after *Modern Healthcare* magazine, a popular trade journal for hospital executives.

Andersen Consulting champions *execution as strategy,* which addresses the idea that creating a compelling strategic vision is but one element of building the future—actually executing that vision is perhaps more important. By executing effectively, an organization can cover up a lot of strategic blunders. A classic example may be Federal Express. The notion that overnight mail should be delivered centrally from one place in the middle of Tennessee is kind of ludicrous on its face, yet FedEx has executed superbly, and the strategy, however loony it might sound, has proven to become a mainstream of American communication.

Community-based integrated systems, whether virtual or actual, were at their core a good idea. They were a good idea poorly executed or not executed at all. There remain a few pioneers, such as the Henry Ford Health System in Detroit, that are still committed to this model. More organizations need to recommit, not to hospitals turning primary care physicians into indentured servants, nor to developing badly run provider-sponsored HMOs, but to hospitals and health systems working collaboratively with physicians and payers to build seamlessly coordinated systems of care for the communities they serve.

Vertical integration was the megatrend that everybody in health care talked about in the early 1990s, but in fact the real integration megatrend has turned out to be horizontal integration among health plans and hospitals (and to a lesser extent among physicians). For example, Aetna U.S. Healthcare bought other HMOs, including Prudential, New York Life's NYLCare, and U.S. Healthcare (the latter for some $9 billion). As the health plan and hospital markets each concentrate horizontally, they have increased the feasibility (if not the likelihood) of more exclusive and more vertically oriented virtual relationships among the various actors in the health system. So one cannot rule out there being greater vertical integration in the future. Nevertheless, the promise of managed competition, which was that these entities would be exclusive, oligopolistic, and vertically integrated, has really not materialized in most markets. Partly this is due to physicians' distrust of both the managed care industry and hospitals and to their desire to hedge their bets by broadening their affiliations beyond one specific institution. Consumers are equally reluctant to commit to one tightly focused network. Part of the backlash against managed care, as we will see in Chapter Five, is really driven by consumers' desire to have access to the broadest possible range of specialists. In the United States, choice is the surrogate for quality.

The Role of For-Profits and Not-for-Profits

American health care is largely a nonprofit enterprise. The rhetoric of the privatization of American health care holds that health care in general and hospitals in particular are increasingly operating on a for-profit basis. In fact, the for-profit hospital sector has accounted for a relatively constant share (about 15 percent) of hospital beds over the last twenty years. But although the for-profit hospital sector has held a relatively constant share over time, there has been a cycle of various consolidation plays. Many of these consolidations were orchestrated by Thomas Frist (founder of the Hospital Corporation of America) and his colleagues to consolidate the same hospitals over and over again, in successive corporate roll-ups. The cycle sweeps investors up in the acquisition phase of accumulation, in which hospitals are acquired, only for these schemes to fall apart and fall out of favor with Wall Street because real, sustainable profits cannot be delivered. After the companies collapse or falter, struggling hospitals are divested and new hospital chains are re-created from the rubble of the previous economic play. For example, for-profit hospital chains American Medical International (AMI) and National Medical Enterprises (NME) begat Tenet Healthcare. Hospital Corporation of America (HCA) begat Columbia/HCA. For-profit hospital chains go into turmoil, and new consolidators emerge from the rubble, many of them using capital they accumulated in the previous round of restructuring. It's like a little shell game that moves its location around from corner to corner in Times Square.

To vilify the for-profit sector in health care is to confuse the issue. In large measure, the for-profit sector has brought capital into health care. The most recent financial roller coaster of the physician practice management (PPM) companies in 1998 and 1999 is testimony to that fact. During the growth phase, PPM companies sucked money out of U.S. mutual funds to buy practices from physicians. That money stayed in the health system—albeit used not to deliver any actual care but to swell the coffers of individual doctors who had sold their practices. Those doctors, if they were smart enough, took the money or the shares used to purchase the practice and immediately turned them into liquid cash or, better yet, bought Yahoo! stock. The unfortunate who took payment in stock (or, worse yet, stock options) are underwater. Those who were fortunate enough to liquidate their purchases are now in a position where they can buy their practices back for ten cents or even one cent on the dollar. Better yet, some physicians are simply being given their practices back because these PPM companies have collapsed under their own Ponzi schemes.

It's likely that when the accounting is all done, the net amount of capital brought into health care from shareholders exceeds the amount of capital that has gone out of the system in the form of profits.

Actually, there is less profit in health care than one might think. For example, if we diverted the entire net income stream for the pharmaceutical industry, it would pay for only three or four twelve-hour shifts for the entire health care system. Indeed, in the late 1980s, my colleagues and I at the Institute for the Future were asked to conduct a study on health care opportunities for Chase Manhattan Bank. The bank asked us for a very simple thing: on one sheet of paper, show where all the money flows in U.S. health care, and on another, show where all the profit was in U.S. health care. A simple question, a very difficult project to deliver on. We developed a map of U.S. health care that showed the flow of funds. It was largely drawn from national health expenditure data from the HCFA, and through a few cartographic tricks we tried to portray the way in which money flowed from the payers, through the hands of intermediaries (insurance companies) on behalf of consumers, to the providers. We used the same base map to show where profits occurred in health care. Comparing the two maps was quite interesting: although one could see the flow of dollars through the system, what was important to note was where profit really was and was not evident compared to the level of expenditure. Bear in mind that this study was done in 1988, prior to the ascendancy of for-profit HMOs and prior to the ascendancy of PPM companies, Columbia/HCA, and the rest. In 1988, if one looked at where profit was made in health care, it was concentrated heavily in one sector: the pharmaceutical and medical equipment manufacturers. They not only made profits but also had a structural interest in declaring those profits to the community, because of their for-profit and publicly traded status. Our clients at Chase were somewhat astonished by this. They saw that there was very little profit either on the hospital side, which wasn't doing particularly well at the time, or on the insurance side, given that the vast majority of insurance companies were at the bottom of the health insurance underwriting cycle. At that time there were very few for-profit conversions among the Blue Cross–Blue Shield plans, and for-profit managed care organizations like PacifiCare and United Healthcare were at the edge, just at the beginning of their massive takeoff in popularity.

Probing this question further, our clients at Chase asked, "Well, who else really does well economically in health care?" Our response was two groups: specialist physicians who enjoyed excess incomes relative to the global incomes of specialists, and most not-for-profit hospitals, in the form of accumulated surpluses and operating margin. None of these profits are declared as profit in the Wall Street sense.

Perhaps the greatest confusion in health care is around the not-for-profit sector. In my presentations, I frequently joke about a fictitious religious hospital chain I call the Sisters of Sustainable Competitive Advantage. The chain is meant to represent both the religious and nonreligious community hospital–based systems, many of which are doing very nicely, thank you, and which cloak themselves in high-sounding mission statements and value statements around community service but operate in much the same way as a for-profit business. Their leaders use the language of business; they talk in terms of business values; they are, in many instances, behaving like CEOs of Fortune 100 companies. This puts these leaders at odds with the rhetoric of community service and the vision and values of community healing that are supposed to be the fundamentals of their institutions. Clearly my joke is an unkind generalization, as there are obviously many, many well-meaning and well-intentioned leaders in the U.S. hospital system. Nevertheless, it is increasingly the case that the sheer scale of these institutions, their economic clout, and the importance attached to their economic survival have made these nonprofit institutions big business. They walk a fine line between "No money, no mission— we cannot serve if we don't survive" and being focused exclusively on profitability, growth, and financial success.

The not-for-profit sector should be different in its orientation and requires and deserves special treatment in terms of taxation. But the for-profit players often refer to their nonprofit compatriots as the nontaxpaying sector. There's a legitimate beef in that remark: If an institution is not differentiating itself from its for-profit competitors, does it really deserve to be given tax breaks? The key differentiation is not in the mission statement of the hospital nor the vision they espouse, but in the behavior of those institutions in the community. It is more important for a not-for-profit institution to *behave* as if it's not-for-profit than to hide behind high-falutin' vision and mission statements. These behaviors must be tangible for the community: for example, demonstrating willingness to provide care to those who are vulnerable and have no means of providing the care for themselves. But the activity also has to be measurable. The move toward measuring community benefit in a systematic way by those in the Healthier Communities movement is an advance. Hospitals and health systems are placing themselves under greater scrutiny rather than simply engaging in financial shenanigans by merely claiming that foregone profit margin was in some sense a community benefit. The institutions are being more careful in their accounting of the total benefit that communities derive from their not-for-profit status.

The Challenge of Regional Diversity

The United States is a big country. If you were to travel as I have over the last fifteen years through most of the major metropolitan markets in this country, you would be deeply struck by the enormous variation in local health care markets. We are not all on an inexorable march to look like San Diego or Minneapolis. The actors are different; the starting points are different; the trends may be similar, but the trajectories are different. Some places have capitated medical groups, others don't and are unlikely ever to develop them. Some places have a lot of Medicare risk contracting, others very little, and again these differences will likely persist.

The range of markets is quite significant. In an Institute for the Future report conducted in 1994, my colleagues and I identified "six Americas," but we could as easily have described sixty or six hundred Americas. The six we described were in the four major regional markets of the United States: the West Coast, the Northeast and Atlantic seaboard, the South, and the Midwest. These markets each had their own particular set of characteristics:

- The wild, wild West was dominated by large medical groups interested in capitation as a form of reimbursement, by high penetration of HMOs, and by high penetration of Medicare risk contracting.
- The South was the Richard Scott Memorial Zone, named for the former maverick CEO of Columbia HCA. This zone was the hotbed of for-profit hospital chains, such as Columbia/ HCA, as well as PPM companies, such as Phycor.
- The Northeast was dominated by the power and prestige of the academic medical centers. In the Northeast (Boston in particular), academic medical centers have disproportionate clout in both the managed care market and in the provider sector compared to other markets, such as California, Arizona, and Oregon, where the academic players are just one of many institutions in the community.
- The Midwest states we described as the PHO zone, because here the markets tended to be focused on nonprofit community hospitals and eager to engage in experiments like physician hospital organizations (PHOs), which were efforts to preserve the status quo.

Each of these markets has a different key actor or different initial condition or different evolution. We also identified two outliers within these regions:

• Florida, which unlike most of the South, had a very high penetration of both elderly people and HMOs. The concentration of elderly retirees has made Florida a mecca for health care services, both good and bad. Utilization levels, concentration of specialists, and concentration of medical charlatans has been greater in Florida than in any other place on the planet. The Florida market has seen waves of change, and the history of for-profit managed care, in particular, has been a fairly sorry one. For example, Florida has a disproportionate concentration of HMOs that fail to receive accreditation from the National Committee on Quality Assurance (NCQA).

• The other anomaly is Minnesota and, to a lesser extent, its neighbor Wisconsin. Minnesota is socialism right here in the United States. Although it is the birthplace of HMOs and the headquarters of United HealthCare, the leading commercial HMO, Minnesota bans for-profit models of health care. It is a state with a homogenous population, with a high penetration of managed care, but no for-profit HMOs. It has a political legacy and community focus much more analogous to the prairie states in Canada than to the states in rest of the region.

To repeat, the point of the Six Americas analysis was not to predict that everyone would end up looking like California but to highlight regional diversity and that different states have different actors who rule the roost.

Although the trends were similar across U.S. markets and the rise of managed care is a megatrend, the way in which these trends will play out in various states and various metropolitan markets is very different depending on the actors. For example, Wisconsin has a high penetration of managed care (around 40 percent) but a very low penetration of Medicare risk contracting. This discrepancy is largely a function of low adjusted average per capita cost (AAPCC) rates, that is, the amount of money an HMO receives for each Medicare recipient each month. (Until recently this was set at 95 percent of the average costs of a fee-for-service Medicare recipient in that county.) Low AAPCC rates have proven an impediment to the penetration of managed Medicare in states like Wisconsin. Other examples of this regional diversity are such states as Maryland and New Jersey, which have a history of rate regulation in the hospital sector; this regulation has significantly affected the penetration of capitation and discounted managed care reimbursement for hospitals and physicians. Similarly, Pennsylvania had a long tradition of low uninsured rates, high health care costs, and an insurance market dominated by the Blues. As players like U.S. Healthcare made significant inroads in this state, the closed marketplace unraveled and providers became exposed to more aggressive managed care pricing.

The challenges of change we have examined—differentiating health from health care, finding a theoretical framework for health care, making community-based integrated systems work either virtually or actually, resolving the confusion and fuzzy thinking around for-profit and not-for-profit status, and responding to the challenge of regional diversity—are in the main uniquely American issues. Through the late 1980s and the 1990s, managed care has been the rubric for dealing with these challenges of change. It was thought that the tension between health and health care could be resolved through managed competition and the rise of capitation. In a managed care world, it was believed that the combination of capitation and integrated systems could align the incentives of providers, patients, and payers. In such a world, managed care could be for-profit or nonprofit and accommodate both the market and community service. It was hoped that managed care could evolve across the country, with one market progressing through a set of logical stages to a better future. Managed care and managed competition were supposed to resolve these particular challenges of change, but as we enter the new millennium, managed care is under assault. What happened?

Chapter Five

The Road to Managed Care

Like all health systems around the world, the U.S. health system is struggling to develop a sustainable compromise among cost, access, quality, and security of benefits. And, as we have seen, there are some particular challenges of change that are specific to the United States. It is in this context that the United States has focused on a unique response: managed care. Although the managed care marketplace is currently unpopular and many of the organizations are in disarray, we have no serious alternative. We don't do government, so megagovernment programs are unlikely to be the answer. We have to build on managed care.

A key step to improving managed care in the new millennium is to understand how we got to where we are. This chapter reviews the four phases in the development of managed care and highlights the current challenges facing the industry.

The Four Phases of Managed Care

During the fifty years of its evolution, managed care has gone through four specific phases. Reviewing these phases will remind us that although managed care has indeed evolved, we must recognize that it is still a work in progress.

Phase I: Radical Reformers

The first phase of managed care, up to the late 1970s, was the phase of the radical reformers. These were the traditional group and staff-model HMOs created by lefty, ponytailed doctors from

Harvard and Stanford who rejected fee for service as a basis for medical practice and embraced prepaid group practice as the model around which health care should be organized. Originally sponsored by large employers, as in the case of Kaiser; by academic institutions, as in the case of Harvard Community Health Plan; or by community organizations, as in the case of Group Health of Puget Sound; these pioneering health plans focused on providing an integrated health care product to working people at a reasonable cost to both the employers and the employees. In this model, physicians would be paid on a prepaid basis, not on a fee-for-service basis, a notion that was particularly antagonistic and threatening to the traditional medical hierarchy. In the 1960s, young physician radicals stood shoulder to shoulder with pioneers of prepaid group practice against the AMA. Now these aging radicals are among the fiercest critics of for-profit managed care, in that they feel that modern, contemporary for-profit managed care has really abandoned the legacy of its not-for-profit forebears.

Phase II: Easy Pickings

Some of the radical reformers who were left-leaning in the 1960s discovered capitalism in the early 1980s, when the for-profit HMOs became a legal alternative. For example, Dr. Robert Gumbiner at FHP was one of the first of the radical pioneers to do HMO conversion, creating a for-profit HMO and the nonprofit FHP Foundation. This was the first of many conversions through the 1980s to create what has become the for-profit managed care industry.

Whether health plans were for-profit or nonprofit, the 1980s was a period of easy pickings. Certainly there was an underwriting cycle, and there were three years of plenty and three years of lean times in the 1980s, just as there had been in the insurance underwriting cycle over the last thirty or forty years. In the main, though, the only requirement to be successful in managed care in the 1980s was that you turn up. Even Kaiser could shadow price against traditional fee-for-service alternatives, thereby making a surplus and pleasing its bondholders and its physicians. Similarly, the for-profit competitors could flourish. Using sophisticated marketing techniques to gather less sick populations in both the commercial insurance market and, in the later part of the 1980s, the Medicare risk market, HMOs became very profitable.

Medicare HMOs had particular commercial success through the late 1980s and early 1990s. Medicare HMOs were established in 1985 but had very limited acceptance among the elderly for the first three to four years, with only one million subscribers (some 3 percent of Medicare recipients) enrolled. Then the combination of aggressive marketing by organizations (such as PacifiCare) and favorable market conditions caused by rapidly escalating premiums for supplementary Medicare coverage made the Medicare risk market take off; by 1998, 16 percent of Medicare recipients were in HMOs.

The success of PacifiCare's Secure Horizons brand demonstrated that HMOs could be not only appealing to the elderly but also extremely profitable. The liberals asserted that this success was attributable to HMOs' cream skimming, that is, picking off the elderly with significantly less health problems. The facts are unassailable in the sense that the reported health status of HMO enrollees under Medicare is significantly less severe than the fee-for-service enrollees. Far less clear is whether or not this situation is the direct fault of Medicare HMOs' marketing practices. In truth, from a marketing point of view you'd have to be an idiot to stumble across the frail, sick elderly in your marketing efforts as a Medicare HMO. The traditional and most effective route for signing up Medicare recipients to HMOs is for seniors to tell other seniors. PacifiCare in particular used this approach, through its Ambassadors Program. Under the program, healthy, well elderly who are participants and big fans of the plan help enroll friends and neighbors in their communities, much in the same way the MCI "friends and family" program works. Without any egregious marketing intent, those ambassadors are going to recruit and encourage enrollment from like-minded future ambassadors. This is a form of "viral marketing" (a term popularized by Tim Draper, the venture capitalist, in reference to Internet marketing strategies).

Similarly, for commercial HMOs, the enormous increase in traditional health insurance rates in the period from 1988 to 1991, coupled with the significant economic slowdown, led many employers to aggressively promote managed care among their employees. In tough economic times few complained, and HMO enrollment spurted.

Success in both the Medicare and commercial segments resulted in a period of growth, prosperity, and significant market capitalization of the for-profit HMO industry, as all of the managed care field flourished through 1994 and 1995.

Phase III: Commoditized Giants

Around the time of the Clinton plan, interest in managed care accelerated, consolidation quickened, and many of the HMOs that were flourishing found themselves in the position of being commoditized giants—behemoths that were undifferentiated from one another and competing only on price. The analogy here is long-distance telephone service. Every night, you get a call from MCI or Sprint asking you to switch from one long-distance program to the other—even though there is absolutely no difference in the market offering, no difference in the price, and in some cases no difference in the leased telephone lines underlying any of the alternative networks. In managed health care, competing HMOs have exactly the same provider network. Employers and enrollees see no differentiation in product, pricing, or customer service to make a consumer, or an employer for that matter, care to switch between one and the other. I have been in five different managed care plans in the last five years in California. I have seen the same doctors over the entire period. The changes have been due to changes in employment circumstances, changes in carrier while I was a full-time employee of the Institute for the Future, or changes in carrier made by my current source of employee health benefits through one of my board relationships. One of these HMOs was so administratively challenged that they failed not only to pay my claims but also to send me a bill for the premium. It was thus a case in which I paid nothing and I got nothing, which is what consultants call a compelling value proposition.

The commoditized giants are finding it extremely difficult to differentiate themselves. They have few new ideas. They are under significant pricing pressures, because of the run-up in medical loss ratios (the proportion of health insurance premiums expended on direct medical care), on the one hand, and because of the stinginess of the Big Ugly Buyers of health care, on the other, who have kept premium increases down. The net result is that health plans have been turned into commoditized giants who lose money. According to *Medical Benefits* magazine, 90 percent of HMOs were profitable in 1994, whereas only 43 percent were profitable in 1998. Over the same time period, margins fell from an average of 2.4 percent profit to a 1.2 percent loss.

The ability of HMOs to price themselves out of this jam is limited because, as we will see later, employers are reluctant simply to cave in the way they once did in the late 1980s. Despite the fact we have a burgeoning economy and a very tight labor market, there is little evidence to suggest that employers can or will easily swallow double-digit percentage rate increases in health premiums. (Rather, as discussed in Chapter Eight, their intention is to shift the burden of these cost increases much more firmly onto their employees, under the guise of empowerment.)

Phase IV: New Paradigms

New paradigms is an expression futurists use when they haven't a clue as to what's going to happen next. We are in that time for the managed care industry. We are in the Land of Oz, where middle-aged white guys are making it up as they go along. They don't have all the answers. Many of them are struggling to keep their jobs in the face of declining profits and the rising negatives in both the media and the marketplace. Despite the rate increases in 1999 that returned many health care plans to profitability, health plans are struggling to find new paradigms that are appealing to their constituencies and their investors. Those health plans that are most successful tend to be playing out a for-profit version of a single-payer system, whereby they simply consolidate in local metropolitan areas so as to achieve economies of scale. Chapter Eight reviews in more detail the strategic dilemmas and future directions for managed care.

The Four D's

We have seen that managed care plans currently are commoditized giants in search of a new paradigm. More specifically, they are struggling with the four D's: demonization of managed care, disintegration of care delivery in response to the demonization of managed care, disappointment in cost containment and in earnings of HMOs, and discovery—their search for a new solution.

Demonization of Managed Care

As a nation, how do we feel about managed care? Not great. According to a Harris poll in April 1999, only 31 percent of the public thought managed care was doing a good job, down from 51 percent as recently as 1997. Managed care is second only to the tobacco industry as the most distrusted. Part of this rising distrust is the result of managed care failing to deliver on its promise of improving quality while reducing cost, but it is also a result of the demonization of managed care—the purposeful trashing of managed care by journalists and others intent on bringing managed care down.

According to ongoing surveys by Louis Harris and Associates, in 1994 a full 60 percent of the American public believed that HMOs helped quality, and only 40 percent believed it hurt quality. Those numbers have reversed in the last five years so that by 1998, the majority (some 58 percent) believe that HMOs hurt quality rather than help it. This shift reflects the growing demonization of managed care.

Journalists (in both the print and electronic media) can take a good deal of the credit for this situation. And when we talk about the role the media plays, we need always to remember what Humphrey Taylor, chairman of Louis Harris, points out: that the media function as a mirror, a magnifying glass, and a prism. They reflect public opinion, they magnify public opinion, but they also distort public opinion.

Journalists are always in pursuit of the big corporate guys who rip off the unsuspecting public to their own benefit, and managed care valiantly stepped in to play that villain's role. Indeed, if it were not for coverage of managed care, *60 Minutes* would be called *30 Minutes*. The real tragedy here is that there has been a lack of the discipline and thoughtful reporting that could place the entire managed care industry in a broader perspective. Journalists must take some responsibility for the mismanagement and miscoverage of both the health care debate and the ongoing managed care debate.

The whipping up of anti–managed care sentiment has really been epitomized by the movie *As Good as it Gets*, in a scene where the character played by Helen Hunt rails against the "[expletives deleted] HMOs." California audiences gave the scene standing ovations because it reflected their HMO experience. (Alain Enthoven of Stanford tells the story of being constantly nagged by friends and associates to go see the movie, and on a visit to Paul Ellwood's home in Jackson Hole, Enthoven and Elwood decided to submit to peer pressure. When the scene of Helen Hunt railing against the HMOs came on, nobody in the audience reacted. Of course, they were in Jackson Hole, Wyoming. There are no HMOs in Wyoming.)

One might go so far as to say that we've seen the enemy and it's Helen Hunt (in her role as representative of the public). The reason is this: we have really not been honest with Helen Hunt. To have all the things that she wants—low out-of-pocket costs and unlimited access to happy, high-quality specialists who have time to spend with patients—is really an illusory goal. Helen wants what she can't have and is not really willing to pay for, and nobody is prepared to tell the truth about those circumstances, least of all the media. Rather, the media use her discontent with health care to vilify the managed care industry—the only institution with the potential to give Helen something of what she wants. (Chapter Eight further examines the role of consumers.)

Journalists also deserve some blame for participating in the demise of the Clinton plan, particularly because they covered the political debate the way they cover all other political debates: as a battle of political power between two sides that each have valid points of view. Journalists were not particularly insightful or penetrating about calling to task poorly founded assertions made by either side in the debate. Covering it as a football game detracted from the validity of certain positions that were predicated on research or that represented long-term agreement among various experts in the field. In particular, journalists participated in the vilification of government-sponsored health care in the trashing of all things foreign, whether it be Canadian or German, and in their coverage of medical miracles gone wrong in the hands of the managed cared industry. The journalistic tradition, analogous to America's dependence on the legalistic tradition of point-counterpoint, often does not yield the truth but rather a balanced view of an unbalanced debate. Covering competing claims as if they were equally sensible may be helpful in building compromise, but it does not lead to better policymaking. Sometimes it leads not to the best of all possible worlds but to the worst.

Yet the mainstream media operate with somewhat of a double standard. They are willing, even eager, to use the video news releases from the pharmaceutical and medical technology industry. The morning talk shows are full of medical technology miracles; they cover the wonders of new drugs and medical devices and technology using the canned television images provided by the industry. More recently the media have been given further conflicting incentives with the enormous explosion of direct-to-consumer advertising; page after page of pharmaceutical industry supplements appear in popular media. For example, pharmaceutical giant Pfizer purchased all of the advertising space in an entire issue of *Time* magazine on the "Future of Medicine." Similarly, Johnson and Johnson purchased the advertising space of an entire issue of *Newsweek*.

One personal anecdote that underscores the media bias against managed care: a producer of a well-respected current affairs television show called me for advice. She clearly was intent on doing a hatchet job on a leading managed care CEO, wanting to cover his excess income and the fact that his organization was taking money away from specialists and vulnerable sick children. I remarked that I thought this was the single biggest cliché in American journalism. The story had been done not only by *Time* magazine but also by countless other journalists who were trying to make the point that managed care leaders were profiting at the expense of doctors and hospitals and their patients. I suggested she might do a story showing that hospitals were having their best year ever (1997), that specialist income had rebounded somewhat, and that there was a significant boom time in the pharmaceutical industry. She had little or no interest in pursuing that story and was somewhat incredulous that such trends were actually true.

The point here is not to berate the media but rather to underscore the fact that the media have played a significant role in devaluing the public's faith in managed care. One part of journalists' motivation for doing so lies in insights they gained during the recession of the early 1990s, when they themselves had been thrust into badly run managed care plans by their large publishing house employers. So they spoke from their own experience and that of their colleagues, but they also reflected the experience of people in the community.

Journalists' demonization of managed care, though flawed, mirrored a fundamental truth: that managed care was intent on limiting access to specialists—that is, on providing more systematic (if one takes the positive view) or constrained (if one takes the negative view) access to specialists in particular. In most of managed care, specialty referrals are managed, whether it is done through gatekeeper physicians in an HMO (such as United HealthCare) or within a single medical group (as in the Kaiser model or in some of the more delegated, capitated models of Southern California). Americans believe that rampaging across the Yellow Pages in search of Marcus Welby is inherently superior to some form of organized system of care. The public's gut reaction is that patient choice is better than having anybody else choosing for them, an assumption that may be grossly incorrect. Indeed, the American public's surrogate for quality is choice of provider.

One of the key results of demonization has been a spillover from the managed care industry into the health care system more broadly. Ongoing focus-group work by the AHA indicates that the American public increasingly perceives that hospitals and physicians and the health care delivery system generally are in it for the money. The public believes that hospitals are less interested in patients than they once were, and sees hospitals in a more negative light than they have for several years. Correlating this with broader survey data of the public, the plight of the hospitals does not seem as extreme as that of the HMOs. As we have seen earlier, in ongoing surveys by the Louis Harris organization with regard to whom people trust, managed care organizations ranked just ahead of tobacco companies. Hospitals, though not in a preeminent place of trust, ranked just behind computers and airlines.

But the findings of the AHA focus group do point to the fact that many in the health care community are unhappy. Nurses, especially, are working in organizations that have been downsized, rightsized, and reengineered, and they have seen their profession radically altered. Instead of being the coordinated, caring profession, nursing has become just one of the cogs of the wheel of care delivery in a reengineered health care environment. Nurses are certainly not happy campers, and they are communicating this discontent to the community in which they are involved.

Similarly, physicians act like spin doctors, putting a negative spin on their HMO experience. My own physician, a very distinguished former chief resident of Stanford who doesn't know what I do for a living, posts on the walls of his treatment room some of the best anti-HMO cartoons I've ever seen. In so doing he is communicating to me and to all his other patients his distrust of the managed care monster—"the goddamn HMOs that limit specialty referrals." His attitude has an impact on his patients' perceptions. Physicians have long had an impact on how patients feel about both their own health and their health insurance, and clearly the provider system also has played a part in the demonization of managed care. In large measure, the discontent of nurses and doctors with managed care is aggravated by the gap between hospital staff and their leadership regarding many of these issues. Often hospital staff don't understand why change has occurred and certainly are unhappy about what the changing environment has meant for the pressures they face on the floor and the quality of their day-to-day work life.

Whether they are reflecting on real experience or are whipped up by the media or by discontented providers, Americans have become profoundly dissatisfied with managed care. Repeated surveys conducted by the Kaiser Family Foundation and by Robert Blendon and colleagues at the Harvard School of Public Health have shown that the Achilles' heel of managed care is discontent with quality associated with specialty referral. This discontent has sown the seeds of the second D of managed care, the disintegration of health systems.

Disintegration of Health Systems

By *disintegration of health systems* I mean the broadening of networks and the loosening of controls that took place in the mid-1990s in response to consumer pressure and employer pressure whipped up by the media against the managed care industry. The argument was that HMOs were delivering inferior quality because they were restricting patient choice through a fixed subset of providers. The HMOs counterargued that those providers had been selected not only because they had agreed to a discounted fee schedule (in HMO parlance, they were "economically credentialed") but also because they had superior performance in terms of quality across various parameters. That argument had a hollow ring to it in the minds of employers and consumers. Pressure was brought to bear to broaden the networks within HMOs, to allow broader partici- pation of hospitals and more specifically of specialist physicians, and to ease up on the referral process, all so as to prevent con- sumers from responding negatively.

Broadening the physician network had a positive impact on many of the HMOs that were already operating under what is often called the "consumer lite" model. *Consumer lite* refers to the enrollee's ability to select physicians from a much broader panel than in the typical HMO, without having to go through an elabo- rate referral process. United HealthCare and Oxford Health Plans were key pioneers of consumer lite. The Oxford case is particularly instructive. Their focus on providing a network of high-quality spe- cialists for the benefit managers of picky metropolitan New York companies made for a compelling HMO value proposition. Oxford was attracting a relatively healthy population of affluent, middle- class households. It was able to offer those affluent middle-class households access to specialists bundled in a way that was con- sumer-friendly. Oxford did a lot right, but the company's experi- ence is testimony to the fact that if you broaden your network, if you make access too open, you run the problem of losing control both of your claims process and of your medical management. Even with a relatively healthy population, Oxford ran into trouble. Open networks eventually fall to the dread disease of IBNR. (*IBNR* is an accounting term that refers to expenses that are "incurred but not reported"—claims expenses that have been incurred and that the HMO will have to pay but of which the HMO is not yet aware.) Like unsafe sex for the promiscuous, as networks get looser, the risk of IBNR goes up exponentially.

In every HMO I've come across, there is a battle around the question of loose or tight networks. Over the last few years, the bat- tle increasingly has involved the CEO as mediator between the marketing guy, the medical management guy, and the head of underwriting. The marketing guy reports back to his CEO that his customers—the employers and their employees—want an HMO in which the patient can go to any specialist any time, anywhere, and pay little out of pocket to do so. The medical management head will respond, "But we don't know anything about the quality of those physicians. We don't know what the economic consequences would be of including them in our panel, and we certainly lose leverage in our negotiations with them by diffusing our lives across an ever broadening network of doctors." The actuary simply says, "I can't compute this problem." As is usually the case with this kind of situation in the United States, the result of these meetings has been that the marketing guy won. Networks have been broadened, and HMOs have introduced point-of-service (POS) products that are the most administratively complex HMO products one can conceive of. Remember IBNR. HMOs have very little control. Allowing patients to self-select away to specialist land at a moment's notice defeats much of the purpose and much of the benefit of coordination of care that is inherent in a well-run managed care organization. The problem of IBNR can plague any organization that loosens its network, whether that organization is operating in the delegated, capitated model of Southern California, whether it's a Kaiser model of integrated care, or whether it's a loose network of individual physicians or IPAs.

This disintegration, even though positive as a kind of freedom-fighting element for the patient, has certainly contributed to a lack of control of health care costs and health care utilization. Indeed, experts and leaders in the delegated, capitated medical groups attribute much of their losses to the rise of POS and the defanging of the HMOs by the media and the public. In other words, these organizations couldn't control costs because they had accepted delegated and capitated risk (care of a defined patient population for a fixed per capita fee per month). Due to pressures from their contracting HMOs, they have been forced to allow patients to move out of network on a POS basis when the patients are willing to pay the difference in copayments. Experienced medical groups who once were successful in managing under a capitated budget constraint are now finding it increasingly difficult to estimate the cost of referral out of network and to manage those costs once initiated.

But disintegration can have an upside. Properly managed HMOs can please their customers by increasing customers' freedom. Perhaps one of the leading examples of a true success story in this area is Blue Shield of California. They introduced their Access Plus HMO product with the intention of servicing the market of discontented consumers who were looking for an opportunity to trade up with their own money if they felt they were not receiving appropriate specialty care. Blue Shield's careful marketing analysis closely paralleled the public policy analysis and more macro-level research conducted by colleagues at Louis Harris and at Harvard, and really reflected the discontent the public was experiencing more broadly with specialty referral. But the Blue Shield case is one of a growing number of examples of what one might term *fine-print marketing*. Although it is true that patients are empowered to choose and visit specialists, they are also required to pay a fairly significant copay of approximately $35, and, as the very fine print states, the specialists they can select have to be from within the same medical group with which the patient already works. This approach provides a way for Blue Shield to make sure their patients are not rampaging all over the California health care system in search of another opinion.

The interesting thing about the Blue Shield experiment is that very few patients actually exercise a choice. In various forums, Blue Shield staff have reported that anywhere from 6 to 10 percent of patients actually utilize the provisions of the Access Plus feature. Also interesting is that only approximately half of the patients didn't even know they had an opportunity to utilize the provision. The Blue Shield experience points to a very well thought through marketing position, that of presenting the enrollee with choice, or at least the illusion of choice. This is really at the core of what the public is asking for.

Practically speaking, most humans do not need to have the opportunity to visit every doctor in their state; that would present an overwhelming set of choices. What the public is deeply concerned about is being locked into poor choices. And this concern really has undermined the basic conception of managed competition, which, as we have described, is that you pick a plan (with a restricted set of providers) when you're well, and you live with the consequences of that choice when you're sick. American consumers clearly reject the notion of living in some kind of perpetuity with a restricted set of choices. As circumstances change, they want the ability to skate away to a different waiting room with a different type of provider.

The disintegration of care has occurred not only to network forms of HMOs but also to the more integrated forms like Kaiser and the Henry Ford Health System in Detroit. All of these plans have broadened their networks one way or another, either by using hospitals in the community that were not part of the system prior to this change or by contracting with physicians in the community.

The public insists on choice under the assumption that in preserving choice one preserves quality. It is important to challenge this quality assumption. There is little or no evidence to suggest that consumers get better outcomes by rampaging around. Kaiser and other integrated forms of HMOs receive the highest marks of all from the various accreditation and medical quality review organizations, such as the NCQA and the Pacific Business Group on Health. There's no evidence that tight integration means poorer quality, but certainly there is evidence that the public sees lack of access and lack of choice as negatives from a quality point of view.

To appease a disgruntled public, HMOs broadened their networks, and this in turn weakened and diffused the concentration of the HMOs' negotiating power with the provider networks and limited the HMOs' cost-control capacity. In response, HMOs have been forced to consolidate in the marketplace to gain market share in a local area. With a large local market share, HMOs are able to provide both broad choice and low cost simply by sheer scale; providers have little or no choice but to contract with these new large plans. This strategy is what I have termed *virtual single payer;* we will return to it in Chapter Nine when we deal more in depth with current and future strategies of health plans.

Disappointment in Cost Containment and Earnings

There has been a sharp turnaround in medical loss ratios in the late 1990s, so that instead of making money, HMOs are losing money; and premiums, instead of going down, are heading up again at high single-digit if not double-digit rates. This trend is partly a result of the broadening of networks. Partly it is a result of more expensive medications being used more frequently by physicians under managed care because of the restrictions on their time. It is partly a reflection of the inexorable rise in medical technology and intensity of care for any given disease. It is partly the reflection of the lack of control on rural medical care prices and utilization. It is partly because of society's inability to deal with very dread diseases without doing everything possible (provided there is insurance coverage).

The broadening of networks coupled with increases in the use and costs of new technology has exposed the lack of effective medical management among the HMOs. In turn, the failure to manage medical care had led to deteriorating economic performance through the late 1990s. To combat this deteriorating economic performance, HMOs have been forced to raise rates, and many of the battles over rates have been bloody. For example, in 1998 CalPers, the health plan for California state employees, balked at a double-digit rise in prices from Kaiser, eventually capitulating to some degree and accepting higher rates. The story has been played out across the country, market after market, with various managed care plans and health insurance carriers across all product lines asking for anywhere from 8, 10, 12, and higher percentage rate increases. Whether in regulated states, such as New York, or in less regulated states, such as California, premium rates have been heading up.

In addition to the upward rate trend, there is also increasing potential as we turn toward the millennium through 1999–2000 for there to be continued *rate dispersion*. When the health insurance underwriting cycle is in its compressed phase, rates tend to concentrate around a mean level. In other words, in 1995 through 1997 in California, the difference in premium between HMO and PPO product was relatively low. Similarly, the difference in premium between large- and small-group insurance was relatively low. This tight concentration of prices reflected a highly competitive environment at the bottom of the underwriting cycle. As HMOs seek to return their plans to profitability, there will be greater dispersion in the prices set for these products in the marketplace. Thus small-group PPOs can be expected to be at the high end of the increase, large-group HMO rate increases at the low end of the increase. This is less true in California because of the impacts of rate-banding controls imposed in the legislative reforms of the early 1990s. Generally, across the country, the assertion holds true that small-group PPOs are likely to experience 12 to 15 percent price increases relative to increases for HMOs and other large organizations, which are going to be in the 8 to 10 percentage-point zone. These rates obviously will vary market to market, but this dispersion in pricing could potentially signal a reenergized interest in more tightly integrated care delivery—provided truly integrated care can deliver the goods.

Unfortunately for those who believe that tighter integration might be a positive step, the key question is really whether there is an enduring advantage to integrated care. Alternatively, does the power of large insurers who have sufficient market power to offer broad networks and low cost simultaneously because they can get better discounts from hospitals and physicians overwhelm any attempt by an organization to integrate care more effectively? It would seem that the money is still on the large, powerful player rather than on the integrated system, at least in the short run.

Ironically, we've suckered HMOs into doing the work that in many other countries is done by government—the rationing of health care—and in this country it has been done on behalf of corporations that want to control their health care costs. And now, after suckering them into doing this for us, we are going to regulate them and maybe even prevent them from doing the work we asked them to do in the first place, by requiring that they provide certain benefits to various disease groups. The famous drive-by birthing legislation is just a precursor of other forms of federal and local legislation. That governments are mandating HMOs to do certain things for certain disease groups (such as patients with diabetes, leukemia, or breast cancer) is a very alarming trend. Taken to its logical conclusion, this trend will hamstring not only the managed care industry but also the medical profession to the point where disease-specific legislation will be the only way to change medical practice. These regulatory controls on practice are the medical equivalent of state mandates and are a way for activists, lobbyists, and the provider community that may benefit from legislative changes to shape the flow of funds to their sector of the health care system. If we take a step back and look at these regulatory controls on clinical practice, it doesn't seem to be in anyone's broad interest to make this kind of piecemeal legislation our vehicle for the future. Such an approach seems to undermine the principles of integration and management of care, on the one hand, and the autonomy of providers to make appropriate decisions, on the other.

Discovery: The Search for New Solutions

Managed care is currently scrambling to redefine itself and return itself to profitability, but there is an alarming and worrying lack of innovation in the managed care industry. Those organizations that have been most innovative, Oxford being the stellar example, are the ones that seem to be struggling mightily to get back to a position of profitability. And they certainly do not seem to be using innovation in any way as a source of economic recovery. Rather, they have used more of a back-to-basics and customer-service orientation without really exploring any new paradigms for the industry.

There is a great thirst for change in U.S. health care, yet the managed care industry, which twenty years ago was the pioneer and leader of innovation in health services organization, is now the laggard in terms of innovation in health care delivery. Perhaps we must look beyond managed care for the source of innovation for the future. One possible approach is to look abroad, as the next chapter does, to see if we can find a new paradigm for health care.

Chapter Six

The Global Context

It may be some consolation to Americans to know that health care is in turmoil around the world. In Canada, Australia, Singapore, Taiwan, the United Kingdom, France, or Germany, you cannot escape in the local media some concern about health care crisis, health care chaos, health care reform, health care restructuring. Perestroika in various forms is epidemic in the health systems around the planet. Some in the United States are glibly climbing aboard the global bandwagon—"Well, we all have the same problems"—but that excuse is invalid. Not everybody is in exactly the same boat as the United States. Most countries have been more successful than we have in providing a sensible and compassionate balance among cost containment, access for all of its citizens, quality of care, and outcomes in terms of health status. As Figure 6.1 illustrates, there is no other country in the world spending anywhere near the amount of money we are on health care, nor is any other country expending as great a share of its economy.

There is no developed country other than the United States and South Africa that has a significant proportion of its population uninsured. There is no other developed country in which the rate of escalation in costs and prices has been sustained over a twenty-year period as it has been in the United States. And there is no other country in which the uncertainty and insecurity of health care pervades a large number of its population under sixty-five years of age. Indeed Dr. Steven Schroeder, the head of the Robert Wood Johnson Foundation, notes that the only statistics of comparative life expectancy in which the United States fairs very well is life expectancy at age sixty-five and life expectancy at age eighty.

Figure 6.1. International Health Care Expenditures per Capita, 1997.

Per Capita Expenditures Adjusted for Cost of Living Differences

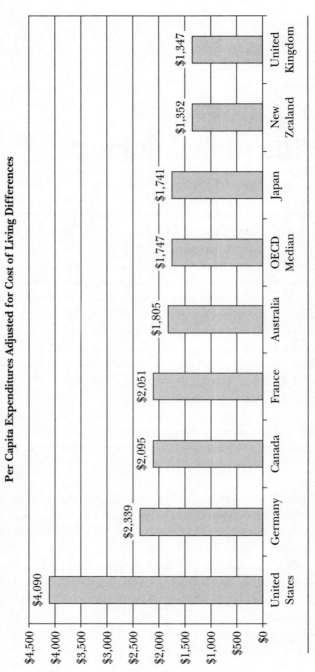

Source: Data from the Organization for Economic Co-operation and Development (OECD); reported by Gerard Anderson, International Health Policy Survey, Commonwealth Fund, October 1998.

He also points out that both age cohorts are the only cohorts in the United States who have universal coverage for their health insurance needs. The good news then is that if you make it to the age of eighty in the United States, you can look forward to living a long and healthy life, just as you would in every other developed country.

It is fair to say that every other developed country in the world has similar concerns about health care. These concerns are about costs and about responsiveness to an increasingly sophisticated public. Cost containment is a pervasive theme in all of health policy, whether the cost containment debate is taking place with health care expenditures at 7 percent of GNP (as in Japan and the United Kingdom), 9 percent of GNP (as in Canada and Germany), or 14 percent of GNP (as in the United States). Most countries, regardless of their different levels of expenditure, have run out of ways to fund their health care system simply through taxation or through their existing premium channels; therefore, they all must contain costs in the future.

There is also increasing concern, particularly in the Western, European nations and in Canada and Australia, about the increased sophistication and demanding nature of the emerging middle classes. Europeans have discovered they're affluent. They are no longer willing simply to accept the social welfare bargain of the postwar period—that bargain being high marginal tax rates in exchange for a reasonable level of security through the social safety net, which made social services like health care available on a socially equitable basis. That bargain had both appeal and economic rationality in an austere postwar environment. As the economies of European countries have expanded and as marginal tax rates have risen to levels approaching 60 percent (or even exceeding that level, as in the case of Scandinavia), countries run out of people to tax. Health care is a major budget item, and therefore high marginal tax rates lead to renewed cost containment pressures and calls from certain quarters, such as physicians and private health insurers, for privatization of the system. These pressures exist in Canada (although Canadians in the main remain committed to preserving a single-tier health system) and in the United Kingdom.

The United Kingdom has a particularly interesting dynamic. Britain's National Health Service (NHS) is the quintessential social- ized medicine system. The NHS is the largest employer in Europe, and the system is the centerpiece of the postwar British welfare state. The legacy of the Thatcher administration and the Conser- vative governments that followed has been to take some of the steam out of the high marginal tax rates that once were applicable in the United Kingdom. The United Kingdom is the most business- like economy of Europe. Even under New Labor, Britain preserves much of the mantle of the free market that emerged in the Thatcher regime, yet under neither Thatcher, Major, nor Blair has there been any interest in wholesale dismantling of the NHS.

A recent international comparative survey, conducted for the Commonwealth Fund by Louis Harris and Harvard University School of Public Health, indicated that satisfaction levels among the English-speaking countries had homogenized somewhat since 1988, when there were wide discrepancies. As Table 6.1 illustrates, at that time Canadians were far and away the most satisfied with their health care system, with the United Kingdom and the United States far behind.

Ten years later, in 1998 Canada's system was less popular than it once was, perhaps as a direct result of the austerity programs put in place in the early 1990s to return Canada to a balanced budget position. Canada's share of GNP going to health care shrank in the 1990s, leading to longer waits for service and growing demoniza- tion of health care in the Canadian media. *Macleans* magazine, Canada's premier news weekly, has run several cover stories on the woes of the Canadian health care system over the last three years, including a cover story about Canadians crossing the border to get Viagra.

In contrast, the British public feel more positive about their health care system than they did ten years ago. This may be a func- tion of recent injections of government financial support for the NHS and a commitment by the Blair government to right some of the perceived wrongs of the more "competitive" policies pursued by the previous Conservative governments. The United States is still close to the bottom of the international totem pole. This low rating may be a function of Americans' high expectations, but it

Table 6.1. International Health Care Satisfaction.

	Rebuild Completely		Minor Changes Needed	
	1988	1998	1988	1998
Australia	17 percent	30 percent	34 percent	18 percent
Canada	5 percent	23 percent	56 percent	20 percent
United Kingdom	17 percent	14 percent	27 percent	25 percent
United States	29 percent	33 percent	10 percent	17 percent

Sources: Harvard/Harris/Baxter Commonwealth Fund, 1988 (Canada, United Kingdom, United States); International Health Policy Survey, Commonwealth Fund, 1998.

also reflects real experiences, particularly among the forty-three million people with no health insurance.

As we have said, the common problems around the world have to do with cost and the inability to pay for health care, on the one hand, and quality and accountability, on the other. The United States is unique in also having significant problems of universal access and insecurity of benefits. Not only are forty-three million people uninsured at any point in time, but a far higher number, perhaps as many as sixty million, experience being uninsured in any two-year period because they change jobs or have bouts of unemployment. Insecurity of health care benefits is very profound in the United States, and this is unmatched in other countries. But with regard to access, there is a growing body of literature and concern in policy circles outside the United States about the inequality of access to health care services based on race, income, and geography even in countries with universal coverage. If you are Canadian and live in Fort St. John in British Columbia, you're going to have very different access than if you live in Vancouver. Similarly, if you are poor and a person of color in the United Kingdom, you are likely to receive less equal care compared to a white person in an affluent suburb. These barriers to care are by no means completely eroded, even in countries with universal coverage.

The Globalization of Managed Care?

Is managed care the global answer to these common health care policy problems? In an attempt to analyze whether there was significant interest in the U.S. managed care model in other parts of the world, Andersen Consulting organized a Health Futures Forum with participants from thirteen different countries. The meeting, which was held in Singapore in 1997, was aimed at identifying the degree to which managed care might globalize.

The Health Futures Forum involved leaders from the U.S. managed care industry and health policy experts from a diverse range of countries, including Australia, Japan, Singapore, Sweden, Norway, the United Kingdom, Malaysia, Taiwan, and the United States. The participants included, among others, Dr. Richard Smith, editor of the *British Medical Journal,* Aki Oshikawa of Stanford University, Dr. Peter MacDonald of the South Australia Health Commission, and Dr. Judy Lim Ming En of Tan Tock Seng Hospital in Singapore.

The forum identified a number of salient points. Although there was significant interest in the concept of managed care, no one around the world really wanted to see a wholesale importation of the U.S. model into his or her country's health system. This attitude reflects a deep understanding on the part of the participants that a country's health care system is the product of the culture and, in particular, a product of the political and economic environment. As we discussed in Chapter One, health care systems reflect fundamental values in the society. Canadians certainly differentiate themselves from Americans based on their health system. In fact, Canadians jokingly refer to themselves as unarmed Americans with health insurance. Even for all their system's recent troubles, they are still deeply proud that no Canadian has to be exposed to the indignity of being uninsured and are quick to point out to their southern neighbors that they spend less money and get more than the average American does for his or her health care dollar. Australians, French, and Japanese are equally proud of their health systems and indeed see the system that has evolved in each of their countries as reflective of their culture.

But the participants were also insightful enough to recognize that their systems were by no means perfect. Indeed, when these health policy experts were gathered in an environment of open debate, they came to the position of recognizing that there is no ideal solution. Although there is a good deal of patriotism and national pride in bragging about one's own health system and trashing America's, the harsh reality is that every health system is an ugly compromise. Every health system has flaws; every health system is in some sense trading off cost, access, quality, service, responsiveness, and universality in order to come to some kind of compromise that meets the utility function and the values of that particular nation.

In this spirit of acknowledging imperfection, the Health Futures Forum was really intended to explore whether or not any of the U.S. managed care tools or concepts were of value in the context of these particular health systems. There were two important findings from the forum. The first, which we have already mentioned, was that no one really wants to adopt in toto the managed care model of the United States. (Particularly obnoxious to some is the for-profit orientation of the managed players.) But, second, there was significant interest in managed care tools and concepts that could be selectively applied and diffused within the health system. This conclusion has been reinforced in individual strategic planning sessions held with leaders in Canada, Australia, and Latin America.

In particular, there was significant interest in tools of *medical management* that might assist the various health authorities, health systems, or health services (however they defined themselves) in managing medical utilization and medical costs. There was also significant interest in *demand management,* that is, in going upstream to the population and identifying ways of intervening in the demand for health care. This may involve empowering consumers with education and providing new information tools and concepts to consumers, such as call-center technology or Internet-based interaction with consumers to deliver information and thereby prevent unnecessary and excess utilization of health services. Additionally, health systems all over the world are thirsty for innovations not only in the delivery of services but in systems to evaluate, monitor, and account for those services so that consumers are better served and payers are served more effectively.

Managed care offers some potential in the areas of medical management, demand management, and systems of accountability for cost and quality. Some of the tools and concepts of managed care could have value globally if they were selectively applied and properly executed to fit a country's unique cultural circumstances.

Execution Matters

U.S. health care industry executives have earned a reputation as pioneers; in many of our policy and management innovations—everything from DRGs in the 1980s to managed care tools and concepts—we seem to be ahead of the curve in theory. However, many visitors to the United States are disappointed to find that we are light on practice and behind on execution. In managed care we have a good deal of interesting ideas—integrated systems, managed competition, the use of electronic medical records—yet there is precious little implementation. And this frustrates visitors who come here to learn, only to find that the much-vaunted theory doesn't really exist on the ground. For example, a group of health care leaders from the United Kingdom visited California in January 1998 under the leadership of Dr. Christopher Ham of Birmingham University. They were in search of a working example of vertical integration that they could hold up as the perfect model. They didn't want to see Kaiser; they had visited Kaiser ten years ago and understood the model well and appreciated its unique achievements. No, they were in search of high-performance virtual integration, with electronic medical records, seamless integration across the continuum of care, disease state management systems—all enabled by cutting-edge information systems. Perhaps needless to say, they left disappointed.

International Health Care System Archetypes

Every health system is unique but it is possible to make generalizations about classes of health systems. A simple taxonomy of international health systems divides the developed nations into four categories: socialized medicine, socialized insurance, mandatory insurance, and voluntary insurance.

Socialized Medicine

The first archetype is socialized medicine, as found in the United Kingdom, Sweden, and Denmark. This form of health care system is one in which the state owns and controls virtually all of the factors of production. It is true that the physicians in Scandinavia and the United Kingdom are not employees per se of the state, but they derive virtually all their income from the state and are under employment contracts (in the case of specialists). The closest approximation to socialized medicine in the United States is the Veterans Administration health system or the military medicine provided directly to personnel by the Department of Defense.

Socialized Insurance

The second archetype is socialized insurance. Canada is the quintessential socialized insurance model, and France and Australia have hybrid socialized insurance models. The basic insurance system in these countries covers all medically necessary services: physicians' services, hospital services, and, to a less universal extent, prescription drugs.

In Canada, prescription drugs are covered for the elderly throughout Canada and selectively for the nonelderly in various provinces. In addition, Canada has a (largely not-for-profit) insurance market for other supplementary health insurance needs, such as long-term care, prescription drug benefits for people under sixty-five, and dental benefits.

In France and Australia, the state does not have a monopoly over coverage for hospital and physician care, and various tiers of supplementary health insurance are available beyond the basic insurance system. Supplementary private insurance covers fees for private practice appointments and covers access to private hospitals. Australia, for example, has a fairly substantial private insurance system and a private sector health care delivery system funded by the private insurance sector.

The closest analogy to socialized insurance in the United States is the Medicare program. Like Canada's system, it is universal (at least for those over sixty-five), comprehensive (although it does not cover prescription drugs), portable across the country, and publicly administered, and it pays physicians on a fee-for-service basis. Medicare is a population-specific version of socialized insurance.

Mandatory Health Insurance

The third health system archetype is the mandatory health systems of Japan, Germany, and the Benelux countries (Belgium, the Netherlands, and Luxembourg). These systems have large, nonprofit health insurance organizations called sickness funds, which provide health insurance for workers, dependents, and other groups, somewhat analogous to the Federal Employees Health Benefits Program. Sickness funds are usually organized around large employers, unions, or work-based associations; those outside the sickness funds are covered by government-sponsored programs. Universality is assured by virtue of the fact that everyone either belongs to some form of sickness fund or is in a government program. These sickness funds coordinate their negotiation with independent, not-for-profit providers and behave largely as monopoly purchasers of health services.

The mandatory insurance system is a close cousin of the purchasing cooperative model operated by the Pacific Business Group on Health (PBGH) in the United States. PBGH is a coalition of purchasers who coordinate rate setting with providers, but for the analogy to be close to the German system, PBGH would have to contract directly with providers, as has been proposed.

Voluntary Insurance

The final archetype is somewhat euphemistically called voluntary insurance. Under voluntary insurance, there is no guarantee of universality. The voluntary nature of the insurance means that there will be some varying proportion of the population left out of health coverage and dependent on receiving care on a charitable basis from religious or other voluntary organizations or on a subsidized basis from local and state government. The U.S. and pre-Apartheid South African health systems are examples of voluntary insurance systems.

Each of these systems has strengths and weaknesses. It is not my intent here to comparatively review or analyze all global health systems; rather it is to point out that the various strengths and weaknesses of these systems are a function of their historical roots and the particular vagaries of the country involved. Even among the English-speaking countries, there is no accord on how health care should be delivered. Canadians, for example, are violently opposed to the incursion of a for-profit hospital sector and to having hospitals and physicians work "both sides of the street." The Canada Health Act of 1984 was a reaffirmation by Canadians of their understanding that if they allowed the wedge of private sector hospitals or of physicians having private practice separate from the Canadian Medicare system, it might undermine the universality of the system. In the United Kingdom, in contrast, the private sector coexists in the form of supplementary insurance. Even though there is no meaningful private sector delivery system to speak of in the United Kingdom, the private insurance enables affluent, covered individuals to jump the queue for less serious procedures, such as an appendectomy. There is no flourishing, for-profit, external system of health care delivery for cardiovascular surgery, for example, because that is incorporated within the National Health Service, and all the key expensive resources are concentrated within the health service sector. In Australia there is comfort with both public and private streams of funding and public and private streams of health care delivery. In every health system, how health care is organized and medical care is delivered has evolved in its own way to account for the values held by the individual country.

The Evolution of International Health Systems

If international health systems were to adopt tools and concepts of managed care, what might those tools be, and how might those systems evolve in the future? The Health Futures Forum focused on how these systems may migrate in the future to some new form.

Socialized Medicine Moves Toward Socialized Health

In the case of systems with socialized medicine, the experts at the Andersen Consulting forum felt that there would be migration toward a model of socialized health; that is, these systems would be recognizing the need to focus on the causal factors behind health, not just on medical care delivery, consistent with a view of health care that is more oriented to population health. A vision of socialized health care also recognizes that the U.K. system, for example, would benefit from the application of the tools of demand management and from some of the incentive tools of capitation. Management lessons could be translated from U.S. capitated medical groups to the U.K. "fundholder" physician groups—medical groups that receive a capitated payment to cover all medical services. Learning from the U.S. experience would yield some positive gain in the U.K. system.

Mandatory Insurance Migrates to a Managed Mandatory Model

Looking at the mandatory insurance systems of Japan and Germany, the Health Futures Forum participants felt that those systems would migrate toward a managed mandatory model in which some of the tools of utilization review would be incorporated into the sickness fund methods of payment. These systems usually operate on a global budget basis. Although the total budgets for hospitals and physicians are controlled by sector, there is little or no aggressive control over the utilization of these services. What this means is that as utilization gets increasingly out of control, prices are continually adjusted downwards to make sure that the overall budgets are not exceeded—what I referred to in Chapter One as the hamster model of reimbursement. But Japan and Germany are conducting experiments in trying to incorporate some of the utilization review and control tools of managed care. For example, sickness funds have signed some deals with U.S. managed care plans in order for these funds to acquire U.S. medical management expertise and utilization review tools and processes. It would be wrong to project successful market entry by U.S. managed care competitors in these markets. Rather, managed care tools and systems will be applied more on a consultative basis within the health sector. Even in that situation we are unlikely to see wholesale global competition in managed care services. However, as global employers seek international solutions from their insurers, across the archetypes we discussed, there is a role for global insurers to play.

Socialized Insurance Systems and Others Become Three-Tiered Systems

The next model that seemed likely to emerge in the future is that of the three-tiered system. Australia clearly is a three-tiered system today and will become more tiered in the future. The largest countries in Latin America—Mexico, Brazil, and Argentina in particular—have three-tiered health systems today. In these countries, there is a basic health system of clinics that serve the very poorest of the population, who may not have mainstream employment and consequently do not pay into the social security systems. The second tier, analogous to the National Health Service in the United Kingdom, is based on social security taxes and provides universal coverage to working people. The third tier is a thriving for-profit private sector system of financing, insurance, and delivery, which caters to the elite of these countries. As the middle tier of socialized health insurance systems moves to privatize, as is proposed in Chile and Argentina, an enormous new market for health insurance services will emerge.

In Australia a significant minority (some 40 percent) participate in the top tier of private insurance; in the Latin American countries only a very small part of the population (less than 10 percent) have access to the private sector. It is in this elite tier that U.S. managed care organizations see a market. Both Aetna U.S. Healthcare and Cigna have made significant health plan investments in Brazil and Argentina. U.S. for-profit competitors are less welcome in Australia, but Aetna has a small position in the emerging New Zealand private insurance market.

Shangri-La Lifecare

A fourth model of transformation was developed that reflected the system of the Health Futures Forum hosts—Singapore. This fourth model of the future was named "Shangri-La Lifecare" by the forum's participants. In the Singapore model, the government has made it mandatory that its citizenry save for their health care needs, through a medical savings account (MSA). Singapore is the best example of this model and is often held up by Republicans in the United States as a key example of how MSAs would look in our country. This is a loony comparison. The MSA in the Republican conception is a voluntary program; it would lead to significant cream skimming—diverting healthier, richer lives to these tax-subsidized vehicles and leaving the traditional Medicare program with a sicker, less affluent population. MSAs work in Singapore because, as Dr. Judy Lim, a prominent health services leader in Singapore, put it at the forum, "We have a compliant population and a strong government." One certainly couldn't apply that description to the U.S. situation.

Singapore succeeds because it has a strong and inexpensive primary care system, albeit one paid for out of pocket. For a fee of around $20, Singaporeans can access primary care physicians who are well trained and competent. They may be paying out of pocket, but the fee is affordable. There is a strong public health system. The patient's MSA money covers his or her hospital and specialty care costs. The outside observer might think this is a crazy way to design health policy, almost the inverse of what one would want. By asking people to pay for primary care out of pocket, you're limiting their access to that care along income lines. Similarly, by giving hospitals an open checkbook from the MSA, you're asking for egregious pricing practices among the hospitals. Despite these valid concerns, it seems that the Singapore system works for Singapore, and indeed the country spends less than 4 percent of its GNP on health care.

Part of the reason this system works is that Singapore is demographically advantaged: very few Singaporeans are over sixty-five. The country also isn't subject to enormous population increases, unlike other neighbors in South Asia, so it has a relatively controlled and youthful population. The tightly controlled society enjoys very low crime and substance abuse rates.

Once Singapore begins to experience the rapid aging of the population that has occurred most recently in Japan, the country cannot expect to hold its costs in line. The population, as it ages, will require more sophisticated and expensive medical care, and the system may start to feel greater pressure. Nevertheless, the lessons for the rest of Asia about ensuring individual access to health care by mandating a savings program dedicated to health has some translatability to other emerging economies in the region.

Lessons for the United States

Although global health policy comparisons have informed U.S. health policy to some extent, U.S. policymakers are uncomfortable looking abroad because what they see in other places is often in conflict with U.S. values and preferences. However, the experiences of other countries reinforce two key lessons about the role of government. First, there is no such thing as voluntary universal coverage. No country has assured coverage for all its citizens without a government mandate. In the United States, we undermine our ability to improve the health coverage situation because we resort to incrementalism—small steps toward expanded coverage rather than reform based on the value of universality. In so doing we often make the situation worse. For example, legislation in California and other states, in an attempt to rationalize the small-group insurance market, created controls on premiums so that they cannot rise beyond a certain band of rates. The result of this approach has probably been to shift up the mean of rates, therefore pricing certain small businesses out of the market. In this way, U.S. health policy manages to shoot itself in the foot. If we are to have universal coverage, the federal government will have to mandate that individuals or their employers purchase health insurance.

The second lesson is that the other countries around the world have had much, much greater success in containing costs from the top down than we have had in the United States through our use of competitive models. The slowing in the rate of health care costs in the mid-1990s that was attributed to managed care was small and short lived. Taking the much longer run view of health care cost containment in the developed countries—looking at the period from 1970 to 2000—yields a different view. Over that thirty-year period, the U.S. record for cost containment is really abysmal. Many countries, Canada included, started off in 1970 expending around the same share of GNP on health. The United States diverted sharply from the experience of other countries, particularly in the 1980s when Canada, Germany, and the United Kingdom applied successive waves of cost containment to meet the escalation of an inflation-ridden 1970s. The lesson here is that macromanagement of health care costs works.

Using global budgets can control costs, but the instrument is a blunt one, and it is becoming apparent around the world that simply applying that blunt instrument as a mechanism to contain cost cannot continue indefinitely. Successive waves of global budget cuts have eroded confidence in health systems around the world, including Canada and the United Kingdom, and there is a sense that you can't simply budget-cut your way to greatness. A climate of permanent constraint leads to a growing sense of malaise and lack of morale in the health system. It's tough to attract the best and the brightest into the health system when all they have to look forward to is doing more of the same with less.

Universal coverage through government mandate and global budget constraints has achieved a lot in health care around the world. But everywhere this system of structured conflict between government and providers shows signs of wear and tear, if not outright collapse. Healthcare is culturally defined. It is a product of politics, economics, and policies that reflect basic societal values. Latin Americans believe in tiering, Canadians do not. No country has the perfect compromise, and each country develops a system that reflects its own values. In the United States we don't believe in government the way most other countries do. We will have to find our own way: a way that is compatible with American values and culture.

Chapter Seven

| Big Ugly Buyers

Purchasers of health care—what I call the Big Ugly Buyers—flexed their muscle in the 1990s. Indeed, over the last twenty years the big buyers of health care have been on the ascendant. Large employers started to join together in purchasing coalitions in the 1980s, and the movement to consolidated purchasing really accelerated in the recession of the early 1990s, when benefit managers were forced to consider new options for reducing health care premiums. Throughout the 1990s both the public and private sectors have become more demanding. The combination of escalating premiums and the global recession of the early 1990s made purchasers much tougher.

Although the shift from defined benefit to defined contribution is well under way, certainly limiting the exposure of the mainstream payers in health care, it would be wrong to suggest that the Big Ugly Buyers will disappear over the next decade. Consumers, particularly the elderly, will never fully pick up the burden that is currently carried by business and government—more than two-thirds of all health expenditures. Consumers are likely to absorb more in the way of costs, but in the aggregate, their outlay will not in any way approach the burden on the Big Ugly Buyers—mega-purchasers who have the capacity to shape the market.

This chapter focuses on three Big Ugly Buyers—Medicare, Medicaid, and employers—and points to the directions they're likely to take over the next decade.

Medicare

Medicare provides universal coverage to the elderly—the most politically active section of the public. Remember that 60 percent of sixty-year-olds vote, whereas 20 percent of twenty-year-olds vote. The elderly have a significant impact on Congress and on the presidency. The seniors membership group, the American Association of Retired Persons (AARP), wields a big stick in Washington. The AARP astutely includes members fifty years old and up, and with the aging of the baby boom, the stick gets bigger.

As we enter the new millennium, Medicare is under assault simply because it is projected that the Medicare program will not be sustainable as the baby boom approaches Medicare eligibility. Currently, the Medicare-eligible age of sixty-five seems far away for the mainstream of the baby boom, but the first baby boomers will turn sixty-five in 2010, only ten years after the start of the millennium. By 2010, Medicare is unlikely to be bankrupted, because the majority of baby boomers will still be in their prime earning and taxpaying years. But after 2020, when the mainstream of the baby boom reaches Medicare eligibility, the picture will change dramatically. By 2030, the peak of the baby boom will have passed into the Medicare system, and this demographic shift, from 2020 to 2030, explains the enormous anticipated jump in enrollment in Medicare.

In 1990, only 12.3 percent of the population was eligible for Medicare. By 2010, that percentage will rise only to 12.9 percent, but by 2030, the share will rise to 19.9 percent. In pure beneficiary terms, the number of elderly beneficiaries is likely to increase from 33.7 million in 1997 to only 36.8 million by 2007. The rise from 1997 to 2017 is from 33.7 million to 47.5 million.

Medicare will increasingly become a program of disabled beneficiaries, not just the elderly. In fiscal year 1997, 87 percent of all Medicare beneficiaries were elderly and about 13 percent were disabled, including those with end-stage renal disease. Medicare beneficiaries with disabilities are expected to grow to almost 16 percent of beneficiaries in 2017, adding a further 8.8 million enrollees to the 47.5 million who are elderly, to a total of 56.3 million enrollees by 2017. These forecasts are based on increases in life expectancy and on the aging of the demographic pyramid that is already in the pipeline.

Medicare Risk Contracting

The key change in the Medicare program that has taken place over the last decade has been the growth in Medicare risk contracting—that is, seniors joining HMOs. Medicare risk contracting was enabled by legislative changes in 1985 allowing seniors to enroll in HMOs, provided the HMOs offered as least as good a benefit package as the fee-for-service Medicare program. In practice, HMOs offered seniors a much wider benefit package, including lower copayments and deductibles as well as coverage for prescription drugs. The proportion of Medicare recipients in the Medicare risk program has grown from approximately 5 percent in 1988 to 15 percent in 1998. The rapid growth in the late 1980s is attributed to aggressive marketing by PacifiCare and other for-profit health plans that embraced Medicare risk as a key managed care market segment. But the growth also reflects acceptance by the Medicare recipients themselves of a superior value proposition (to use the consulting term): the HMO industry was capable of providing both prescription drug coverage and reduced out-of-pocket cost sharing, both of which were popular with patients, all for the basic Medicare premium.

This growth in Medicare risk has transformed many managed care markets, such as Arizona, Colorado, Oregon, and California; in certain places, such as Portland, Oregon, and Riverside County in California, as many as half of all Medicare recipients are in HMOs. Most states have not seen this degree of penetration of Medicare risk; for example, by 1998, Arizona and California had approximately 40 percent of all Medicare recipients in HMOs, compared to 15 percent nationally. California alone accounts for over a third of the Medicare risk population as of 1998, because of the high AAPCC rates and wide consumer acceptance of managed care. Medicare risk grew rapidly from 1995 to 1997 (about 30 percent annually), but it did so disproportionately in the advanced managed care markets. In 1997, 33 percent of the Medicare population had no access to Medicare HMOs, down from 45 percent in 1995.

Part of the reason why Medicare risk has not penetrated more rapidly is that there is nobody to capitate in markets outside the West.

The lack of infrastructure to support Medicare managed care (and by *infrastructure* here I mean medical groups capable of absorbing capitation) has meant that Medicare risk has begun to stall. In addition, private plans withdrew from the market as they encountered losses in 1998. The actions of the HCFA in the Balanced Budget Act of 1997 increased the number of choices available to the Medicare population, including point-of-service HMO and preferred provider organization (PPO) models of managed care. This has further diluted the concentration and likely growth in capitated Medicare managed care. The broadening of choice of managed care model could undermine both the traditional Medicare fee-for-service system and, perversely, the pure capitated risk model. This is because the choice model is likely to create selection effects; that is, the very sickest will remain in fee-for-service Medicare programs, and the more affluent and healthy will select the open-ended choice models.

The Rise of Medicare+Choice

With the Balanced Budget Act of 1997, Medicare expanded the range of managed care choice. The intent of the Medicare+Choice legislation was to broaden the managed care product offering available to the Medicare population and not restrict the elderly to a simple choice between a risk-model HMO or the traditional fee-for-service system. Medicare offered a wide range of managed care choices, including provider-sponsored networks (PSNs)—which are in effect HMOs offered by provider groups. The euphoria over PSNs, however, has been very short lived. As of 1999, the HCFA had received only three applications by PSNs. Part of the explanation for the slow pickup of this policy is that providers have recognized that running an HMO is a very different business from running a hospital. The stakeholders pushing for PSNs—largely the trade associations, the AHA and the AMA in particular—saw PSNs as an opportunity to capture some of the premium dollar flowing to the managed care industry. However, these advocates of PSNs reflect what could be termed the mutual disrespect problem, which is that everyone in U.S. health care thinks that everybody else's job is easy. And in particular, everybody believes they can be an HMO. The truth of the matter is that HMOs have some unique core competencies, such as sales and marketing and underwriting, at least when they're doing it properly. Provider systems, such as hospitals and health systems, simply have had little or no experience with either marketing (certainly to employers) or the underwriting function.

Another significant barrier to the success of PSNs was that the fast-tracking of PSNs from a policy point of view coincided with perhaps the worst period of economic performance for the HMOs. Do you really want to get into a business that loses 3 percent per year? Those hospitals that experimented with HMOs have run into trouble. For example, in Erie, Pennsylvania, St. Vincent's Hospital and Hamot Health System jointly run an HMO. That HMO has struggled financially, and both hospitals regret having started the HMO, although it probably was an appropriate strategic defensive move against incursion from Big Ugly Buyers from out of town.

The Shift from Defined Benefit to Defined Contribution

The recent Medicare commission failed to reach a consensus on the shift from defined benefit to defined contribution for Medicare. Proposals included premium-sharing models, whereby Medicare would pay 88 percent of the median insurance market product for seniors. Alternatively, a pure form of defined contribution has been proposed in which seniors would receive a voucher for a fixed amount. The commission's failure to reach consensus will lead to a new round of counterproposals from the White House and Congress. In the short run modest reform is likely with the benefit package expanded to include prescription drug coverage. In the long run, however, the outcome is likely to be a shift to defined contribution in some form, but this outcome could take us a decade of political wrangling to achieve. As the demographic data show, we have time; we can postpone real policy change for a decade. The question is, will we ever have this opportunity for major Medicare reform again—when the economy is in strong shape and the government budget is in surplus?

The proposed risk-adjustment modifications are an essential part of the overall policy of Medicare+Choice. Absent risk adjustment, there would be even more problems of cream skimming and adverse selection within the Medicare+Choice program. Can we design a choice program that won't unravel in a spiral of adverse selection? Can we add prescription drug coverage and long–term care without breaking the bank or alienating the powerful prescription drug industry? Will the managed care industry hang in there? Is Medicare managed care in whatever form an attractive enough business that would allow the players to make a reasonable profit? What is reasonable?

Much of the future of Medicare depends on the likely political context during the 2000 presidential election and beyond. If Republicans are in the ascendancy both in the White House and Congress, there will be a much greater interest in preserving the elements of both choice and private sector participation. In contrast, if Democrats control both White House and Congress and the traditional liberal bias toward single-payer-type models were to reassert itself, one could imagine a future in which Medicare+ Choice would politically unravel in favor of a single-payer approach, at least for Medicare.

Risk Adjustment

To a large degree the political choice will depend on the success or failure of managed care itself in containing costs. In turn this will require addressing the issue of risk adjustment. (Risk adjustment is the adjustment in reimbursement to reflect the severity of illness and therefore the costs of caring for patients with various conditions.) Similarly, we need to address the management of the chronically ill from the perspectives of health care delivery and of managed care. We need to create an incentive for more focused management of the chronically ill. Properly designed, risk adjustment could discourage cream skimming, encourage providers and health plans to be much more rigorous in their management of specific cases, such as cancer, and provide an incentive to look after those patients in a more cost-effective way than the current fee-for-service model.

The likely consequence of increased choice, unless risk adjustment is addressed, is for an increase rather than decrease in overall Medicare expenditures. Data from the HCFA indicate that on average the enrollees in Medicare managed care tend to be less sick. But HMOs currently are paid a fixed proportion (approximately 95 percent) of the average Medicare cost per capita in that county. Sicker, older Medicare recipients remain in the traditional

fee-for-service program while younger, healthier recipients gravitate toward various managed care models. This trend is going to
lead to a death spiral in the insurance pool unless risk-adjustment
legislation and regulation is passed to ameliorate these adverse
selection effects.

Risk adjustment is a key weakness in the policy of Medicare
going forward. If the market is going to be used as a vehicle for
managed care, specifically the use of Medicare+Choice or some
variant of that model, then it is imperative that this Achilles heel
of Medicare be fixed. The reason why risk adjustment is so criti-
cally important for the Medicare population and indeed for any
insurance pool is that approximately 5 percent of patients account
for 45 percent of all Medicare costs.

A sick patient can cost the system ten to twenty times as much
as a nonsick patient. If the average person enrolling in an HMO is
less sick as defined by health status, then the HMO will in effect be
cherry picking the healthier population, and, overall, the policy of
allowing patients to choose will be cost-inflationary for the
Medicare program in total.

In an effort to deal with this inequity, the HCFA announced
proposed changes starting on January 1, 2000. Medicare officials
are attempting to redress the imbalance of payments paid to
HMOs. HMOs now receive a fixed payment for each beneficiary;
that payment is adjusted only for a few factors, such as the beneficiary's age, sex, and county of residence. But there is no adjustment at the present time for the patient's medical history. On
average, Medicare pays $5,800 a year for each beneficiary in an
HMO. The new payment system proposes that HMOs will receive
extra payments for beneficiaries who have been hospitalized in the
prior years for specific conditions. The bonus ranges from $1,910
a year for a patient with breast cancer to $24,464 for a person with
AIDS. According to HCFA sources reported in the *New York Times*
(Jan. 16, 1999), the extra payment could be $4,666 for heart attack;
$5,969 for colon cancer; $8,474 for stroke; $12,435 for lung can-
cer; and $13,547 for ovarian cancer. Payments for healthy Medicare
beneficiaries could be reduced as much as 20 percent. Policy
experts estimate that at least 90 percent of Medicare HMOs would
see their total payments cut under this system. Medicare officials
estimate that this new method of payment would save $200 million

in the year 2000 and a total of $11.2 billion over five years. Given that HMOs are likely to suffer financially, it is not surprising that HMO leadership groups are upset about the proposed changes. However, this natural concern really has to be placed in a broader context. Without risk adjustment, the Medicare Choice policy is cost-inflationary for the Medicare program and Medicare risk payments are simply not sustainable.

The question that remains is whether private sector Medicare HMOs are given sufficient incentive to remain in the field. Recently, four hundred thousand Medicare patients were dropped by their HMOs. Such major players as United, Aetna U.S. Healthcare, and Oxford dropped their HMO plans in certain counties; their HMOs could not make money in those counties because the reimbursement payment—the AAPCC rate—was too low to be profitable.

Resolving the problems of risk adjustment for this population has to be a high priority of policymakers, but it has proven an intractable problem over the last several years, both politically and technically. The HCFA has made regulatory commitments to resolve the risk adjustment issue. But the HCFA is so administratively challenged by its "Y2K" bug that implementation of risk adjustment and other initiatives could be delayed significantly.

Although Medicare+Choice is the vehicle for the future, it is questionable whether that vehicle is sustainable in its current form extrapolated out ten years. Risk adjustment is one significant part of fixing the problem for managed care. The other is to identify how to contain costs, particularly for the chronically ill in either the basic fee-for-service program or Medicare managed care.

Medicare Managed Care and the Management of the Chronically Ill

Managed care has not really demonstrated enormous success in managing chronic disease. The early gains from reducing hospitalization have run their course, and now the more complex issue of changing the intensity of servicing of Medicare patients is becoming more of a challenge. Disease-state management (DSM) companies were supposed to be the way in which this issue was resolved. However, DSM was most aggressively pursued by the pharmaceutical industry (and in that case it was really disease-state marketing). Sophisticated pharmaceutical companies used DSM and the vocabulary of DSM to gain influence with managed care organizations, with the intent of getting on the formulary.

As risk adjustment begins to change the flow of reimbursement for those patients with expensive conditions, it will stimulate true disease-state management. DSM companies will offer their services to HMOs in a way that allows the HMO to manage under the budget constraint. For example, in the case of a Medicare recipient with ovarian cancer, a $13,547 risk-adjustment bonus would be paid for that individual. The success of such focused funding streams, however, will depend ultimately on the degree to which some intermediary, such as an HMO, can coordinate the payments and delegate the care to various constituent players. And this could potentially lead to the creation of so-called focused factories.

Risk-adjusted payment mechanisms of this type could stimulate further specialization in health care delivery. The risk-adjustment model that is being proposed would encourage specialization and provide an incentive to focus on improving the care of acute and chronic conditions. But if health care delivery continues to specialize into a myriad of focused care delivery systems—diabetic care centers, cancer care centers, cardiovascular treatment organizations, and the like—there is likely to be a concomitant increase in transaction costs (the costs of coordinating among these different specialty areas), which may overwhelm the savings of specialization.

Similarly, as increasing choice is offered to recipients in terms of types of managed care plans, transaction costs also will increase, potentially making the overall Medicare program more expensive rather than less expensive. Part of the appeal of a single-payer Medicare program as it existed was its extremely low administrative cost: less than 3 percent for the entire program, compared to the 15 percent in most of the private indemnity insurance plans and 20 to 30 percent in managed care plans. In a similar way, the integrated HMOs like Kaiser have the opportunity to integrate and coordinate the components of care. By increasing choice of plans and by increasing pluralism and specialization in health care delivery, the HCFA and the Medicare reimbursement system may be inviting a greater proportion of cost to go to administration of the Medicare program.

Erosion of Retiree Health Benefits

A key issue affecting the Medicare population centers on the future of retiree health benefits in the corporate sector. With the move from defined benefit to defined contribution, there is likely going to be erosion of retiree health benefits. For example, there is a well-publicized case involving Pabst Brewery in Wisconsin; the company was accused of reneging on its retiree health benefit commitment. This is perhaps the beginning of a broader trend toward undoing commitments or restricting future commitments to retirees for health benefits. Indeed, according to a Harris survey of employers conducted in 1998 for the Baylor College of Medicine, 15 percent of employers planned to cut back on retiree health benefits in the year ahead.

The erosion of retiree health benefits is significant in a number of ways. First of all, according to an analysis by Towers Perrin, the employee benefit consultants, in January 1998, approximately 30 percent of Medicare beneficiaries had individual supplemental coverage; 24 percent had group coverage; 15 percent were in managed care; 8 percent were dually eligible for both Medicare and Medicaid because of their income; and 23 percent had Medicare only. The 24 percent with group coverage represent a significant part of the mainstream of American retirees. If that proportion erodes over time because of the withdrawal of retiree health benefits, it will place an additional burden on the Medicare recipients to fund their own supplementary coverage for prescription drugs and copayments and deductibles, either through individual coverage or through enrollment in managed care.

The Critical Gaps in Medicare Coverage: Prescription Drugs and Long-Term Care

The two most important gaps in coverage for the elderly are prescription drugs and long-term care. Costs for institutional long-term care facilities are the greatest financial risk for the elderly: 42 percent of all out-of-pocket costs expended in 1993 were for long-term care. Prescription drugs accounted for 18 percent of the elderly's out-of pocket costs. A third of all elderly have no drug cov-

Table 7.1. Distribution of Medicare
Supplemental Drug Coverage.

Type of Coverage	Total (Millions)	With Drug Coverage (Percent)		
		Primary	Secondary	None
All persons	36.7	61.7 percent	3.4 percent	34.8 percent
No Supplemental Coverage (FFS Medicare Only)	3.0	0.0	0.0	100.0
Supplemental Coverage:				
Medicare HMO	2.5	95.0	-	4.1
Medicaid	4.5	87.8	2.0	10.2
Employer-Sponsored	12.1	83.9	2.4	13.7
Individually Purchased Only	10.6	28.9	7.0	64.1
All Other	1.0	78.5	-	20.1
Switched Coverage During Year	3.0	77.0	3.3	19.7

Source: Health Care Financing Administration, 1998.

erage of any form. As Table 7.1 shows, most of the elderly dually covered by Medicaid, in HMOs, or with employer-sponsored supplementary coverage have some form of prescription drug benefit. Less than a third of those with individual supplemental policies have a drug benefit.

A full 80 percent of the elderly are taking some form of prescription medication at any point in time, whereas only 4 percent of the elderly are in a nursing home. The nursing home burden can be in excess of $30,000 per year, whereas the average total drug expenditure for a Medicare recipient is $500 per year. Surveys show that many elderly believe (incorrectly) that nursing homes are covered by Medicare; in fact, Medicaid (the program for the poor) is the de facto nursing home insurer. Prescription drug coverage is politically popular because drugs comprise a significant proportion of the out-of-pocket burden for the average elderly recipient, and, more important, the vast majority of elderly Medicare recipients use prescription drugs. Finally, long-term care coverage would require a $60 to $70 billion commitment by Congress. It is just too big a nut for Congress to crack, at least for now.

Before the emergence of Medicare HMOs, the elderly relied on supplementary insurance—MediGap—purchased by the individual or provided for the lucky 28 percent of the elderly as a retiree health benefit. The individual supplementary insurance market is a classic example of private insurance market failure. Individual Medigap premiums started to rise significantly in 1995 and 1996. This rise was to be expected given the natural inefficiencies of supplementary insurance and the fact that rationalization in the MediGap market in the early 1990s produced a very bizarre insurance market. The reforms of the early 1990s standardized the individual MediGap market into ten types of Medi-Gap policy—only three of which included drug coverage. This change sent an even clearer signal to beneficiaries that they should sign up for those plans with drug coverage only if they had significant drug coverage needs—adverse selection at its most intense. Premiums will naturally rise for this group over time if such adverse selection continues.

Debate about extending coverage for prescription drugs and long-term care will be part of the process of Medicare reform, although it is a tough political and economic challenge to add these new forms of coverage when the program overall is trying to fulfill the current level of commitments to future beneficiaries. A central issue going forward will be the degree to which Medicare covers *and* controls the costs of prescription drugs. This issue is likely to receive more political attention in the next five years. This situation will be brought to a head by the ever increasing sophistication of new medical technologies and the continued aggressive pricing of pharmaceuticals. (Chapter Ten addresses the coming drug price wars as one of the key emerging issues of health care.)

Medicare may choose to respond to this issue in a number of different ways, anywhere from encouraging drug pricing controls on a national basis to creating national formularies or developing best-price legislation analogous to that passed for Medicaid. But

Medicare has always been reluctant to use the full extent of its purchasing clout. Imagine Medicare receiving bids for inpatient care whereby the top three bidders became the preferred providers in a metropolitan area. Considering that hospitals get 40 percent of their inpatient income from Medicare, most hospitals would be toast if Medicare flexed its purchasing muscle. Drug companies know that too, and that's why they are not exactly delirious at the prospect of a comprehensive Medicare drug benefit. The elderly consume a third of all drugs; if the government paid the whole tab, it might start to question the price.

Medicare has become a political football, but it's being tossed around on a fairly narrow playing field in the sense that the fights of the late 1990s were over minuscule differences between Republicans and Democrats, centering on the degree of cost sharing with recipients. In the long run, the United States must struggle with the demographic bolus of the baby boom coming through after 2010.

The political landscape is made more complex by the Republican paradox: "the market is working, but managed care stinks." Medicare, after all, is perhaps the singularly most popular program among consumers. In Harris surveys, consumers continue to give high marks to the Medicare program. So in a real sense, we are trying to fix a system that—at least in the minds of the public—ain't broke.

Medicaid: The Forgotten Health Program

Medicaid is the stepchild of Medicare. It is a combined program that serves the long-term needs of those who are disadvantaged; supplies supplementary health insurance coverage to the poor elderly, the so-called dual eligible; and is the default policy for long-term care support in this country. Two-thirds of Medicaid recipients are mothers and children in the Aid for Families with Dependent Children (AFDC) program. However, two-thirds of the *cost* of Medicaid is for the blind, the disabled, and for long-term care for the elderly. The average middle-class family who runs into an enormous nursing home burden will tend to spend down its assets and become eligible for Medicaid support of nursing home care. This fact has really been a major impediment to the rationalization of Medicaid. The other structural flaw in the Medicaid program is that it is a combined federal and state program (unlike Medicare, for which there are national standards), which leads to enormous variation in quality, funding, and reimbursement across the country. By delegating more of the burden of Medicaid and welfare reform back to the states, legislators have amplified both the regional diversity and the regional inequity that we are likely to see over the next decade.

On the bright side, managed care Medicaid has actually proven to be an improvement for many Medicaid recipients. Fee-for-service Medicaid, although in theory an open-ended benefit, was in practice a severe restriction on access, because in many states, providers simply would not accept Medicaid patients. So although Medicaid patients had a card that in theory would enable them to go to any provider, their choices were severely restricted. By providing Medicaid recipients access to managed care, states have mainstreamed the Medicaid population more than the traditional fee-for-service system ever did. However, in such states as Tennessee that have combined these experiments with efforts to reduce the number of uninsured, there appears to be chronic underfunding of these programs, at least from the providers' perspective. They feel as though they have been mandated to accept losses for providing care.

In other states, most notably California, more competitive models have been introduced. In California, thirteen counties have had a model of Medicaid managed care in which a county-run system in the public sector competes against a single for-profit or not-for-profit competitor in the community—Foundation Health Plan and WellPoint being the two principal for-profit actors in the thirteen counties in California. There are two key problems with competitive models of Medicaid managed care. First, managed care plans, especially for-profit entities, have no long-term moral commitment to that particular marketplace. Unlike the counties and safety-net providers that are in that business, WellPoint could decide in the next two years not to participate if reimbursement suffers and profitability was not there. Second, analogous to the Medicare program, there is an incentive for Medicaid managed care to market only to those AFDC moms and kids who have little or no comorbidity—just simple normal deliveries and well-baby visits. That kind of marketing is supposedly illegal under the terms of the program; nevertheless, in signing up patients for these programs, the companies could achieve selective retention rates through a number of marketing schemes and by creating barriers to entry.

A key bright light in the Medicaid and safety-net markets is the potential coverage for children under the Child Health Insurance Plan or so-called Kiddie Care legislation. Despite the tremendous appeal of this program and the noble goal of reducing the number of uninsured children (more than ten million), there has been abysmal implementation of this program; only a handful of states had brought on full implementation by the end of 1998. The problem is partly organizational and administrative. It is partly caused by the reluctance of states to spend money to achieve the matching dollars from the federal government. And in California and other border states, the problem partly is a result of anti-immigrant sentiment that made the enrollment process unattractive to legal immigrant families. For example, in California the enrollment forms for the program delved into immigration status in considerable depth, often discouraging many Latino families from availing themselves of the new coverage provisions. However, one of the most significant causes of the disappointing implementation of the Kiddy Care coverage is simply that children have not been the central focus of policy either in health care or in any other arena.

A key part of the child health initiative is to encourage children to receive care in a more preventive mode. Children are disproportionately uninsured, so extending coverage to kids will go a long way to ameliorating some of the problems of the uninsured and the negative long-term health consequences of inadequate levels of immunization and lack of primary care for children in the early stages of development. Indeed, Fraser Mustard and his colleagues at the Canadian Institute of Advanced Research have shown over the years that the single most important intervention that can be made in the health status of communities is investment in early childhood development, broadly defined to include child care, family leave policies, preschool and elementary education programs, and effective parenting. This investment is not simply in health care; more important, it is in education, child care, and other forms of social support for children, which inculcate behaviors that promote health and provide a nurturing environment for children. Investment in early childhood development will eventually lead to higher levels of education, economic success, and overall health in the future.

Employer-Based Coverage: Where Do We Go from Here?

One of the key changes that has taken place in the last decade is the erosion in the proportion of employers providing health insurance. This change has been a major contributing factor behind the rise of the number of uninsured. A full 80 percent of the uninsured are working people or their dependents. A survey by Jon Gabel of the Health Research and Education Trust in conjunction with the Kaiser Family Foundation found that the proportion of large firms (those with more than two hundred employees) offering health insurance dropped from 67 percent to 64 percent from 1996 to 1998. The erosion of coverage is even more significant in small business, from 52 percent to 49 percent. This trend in small business indicates that the ranks of the working uninsured will continue to increase. A full 61 percent of all uninsured workers are in firms with fewer than one hundred employees, and 47 percent are in firms with fewer than twenty-five employees.

Contrary to popular opinion, there are uninsured workers even in large firms—24 percent of all uninsured workers are in firms with more than one thousand employees. This is particularly alarming because we designed U.S. health policy in the 1960s as if everybody worked for the Fortune 500. The Fortune 500 employs less than 10 percent of the labor force—a number that is going down rather than up. The policy of tying the average American's health insurance to employment is one that does not really fit with the so-called new economy. Increasingly, people are working in part-time jobs or on a contingent, flexible basis. They are unlikely to stay with the same firm for many years. As more and more people work in a fluid way, be they self-employed, consultants, part-time workers, or temporary workers, tying benefits and health care coverage to full-time employment becomes a more and more difficult, if not ludicrous, way to organize health insurance coverage.

Jon Gabel's survey shines light on one of the great mysteries of employer-based health insurance: the underwriting cycle. This is the mythical three years of famine and three years of plenty enjoyed by the health insurance industry. This is a cycle that even the actuaries don't fully understand. (The best will tell you it is caused by the systematic overestimation of the success of cost containment by the actuaries and the subsequent overreaction in rate setting.) The survey showed that premium increases in 1998 were 5.2 percent for small firms (compared to only 1.8 percent in 1996), and 3.3 percent for large firms (compared to 0.5 percent in 1996). If we follow the underwriting cycle, rate increases are likely to be around 8 to 10 percent in the 1999 to 2001 period, as the HMOs try to dig themselves out of the financial hole they fell into during the 1995 to 1998 period.

Gabel's survey confirms the shift to managed care lite, with PPO and point-of-service HMO plans being the beneficiaries in the small- and large-group markets. For example, Gabel found that "firms dropping conventional coverage tend to move to PPOs, while employers dropping HMO coverage opt for point-of-service (POS). Point of Service plans are HMOs where the enrollee has the right to go out of network for care if they pay the higher co-payments and deductibles involved. In fact the largest shift in market share between 1996 and 1998 occurred in the percent of workers in small business who are covered by a POS plan—30 percent in 1998 compared to only 7 percent in 1996."

The Rise of Managed Care

Ten years ago, few would have predicted that the vast majority of U.S. workers would today be covered through some form of managed care. Even among small business, the last bastion of indemnity insurance, only 13 percent of insured workers have conventional indemnity insurance (down from 27 percent in 1996), and the rest were in some form of managed care.

Major employers, such as AT&T, Xerox, Hewlett-Packard, and General Electric, were the first to be active in pushing managed care during the last recession. Indeed, if one looks at such leaders as General Electric, they have provided incentives and done all the right things to move almost all their employees into some form of managed care. As a response to escalating health premiums, this shift to managed care helped keep the employers' health cost relatively flat through the 1990s. The question now becomes, What do they do for an encore? The next battleground for those advanced employers is to move to a defined-contribution model. They have encouraged their employees and retirees to move into HMOs and other forms of managed care, and they are now aggressively moving to limit and cap the long-term commitment to those employees, be they retirees or regular workers. This shift from defined benefit to defined contribution is most advanced among the most sophisticated in the benefit world, such as CalPers and GE; however, more and more employers are moving in this direction. According to a study conducted in 1998 by Louis Harris and Associates for the Baylor College of Medicine, 52 percent of employers said they would be moving their employees from defined-benefit to defined-contribution models.

Another area where the shift from defined benefit to defined contribution could gain momentum is in small businesses, which historically have not been particularly aggressive in managing health benefits. A significant change in the small business market is the emergence of professional employee organizations (PEOs). PEOs are employee leasing companies that take on all the hiring, firing, and benefits administration tasks on behalf of their customers—small business owners. This model has two benefits. First, it centralizes routine administrative and back-office functions within the PEO, freeing the individual entrepreneur from having to create a human resource infrastructure. Second, by leasing employees the individual entrepreneur can have very different benefit and pension structures from those people working in their offices.

Until recently, the employee leasing business was highly fragmented and focused on very small firms—the average number of employees per client being around eleven. This is in contrast to the more sophisticated temporary help and staffing companies, such as Manpower, Kelly, Interim Services, and Robert Half International, which have grown into multibillion-dollar organizations by providing flexible staffing solutions to large corporate clients.

In 1997, a significant change occurred: sophisticated service players, including CNA Insurance, ServiceMaster, and Nova Care, made aggressive moves into the PEO market through acquisition, consolidation, and rapid increases in investment. Each of these three companies now have PEO businesses with well in excess of $1 billion in sales as of 1999. They present an opportunity to become new aggregators of lives; the aggregation of many small businesses into a pool for purchasing health benefits is analogous to the kind of model that Calpers has built for state employees. Such aggregators have the potential to behave as Big Ugly Buyers. PEOs' market clout is building rapidly in states like Texas and Florida. They will likely have a major impact as a Big Ugly Buyer of small-group insurance when their market share reaches 15 to 20 percent of the small-group market.

Employers' Health Costs Rise Again

The fundamental question for employers of all sizes going forward, however, is how to deal with double-digit premium increases, and the answer has come back loud and clear: pass the burden on to consumers. Employers have done managed care. They have done POS. There seems to be little interest among employers in expanding their commitment to tight managed care; instead they're looking to transfer the burden to consumers as a means of solving their own economic problems.

This response will prove to be a very shortsighted one because, although it is fashionable to talk of empowerment, employees will soon realize that empowerment means paying more out of pocket. And making employees pay out of pocket does not necessarily enable them to strike better bargains simply because they have a reason to pay attention. (No, Doc, $5,500 for the prostatectomy is way too much. I'll give you $4,500. Take it or I walk.")

Indeed, part of the success of managed care and the Big Ugly Buyers of health care has been to significantly reduce hospitalization costs and physician fee structures through the magic of oligopsony (the concentration of buying power). Individual consumers are unlikely to achieve a similar saving. Therefore it is likely that consumers will turn back to their employers for help in negotiating rates and in ensuring that they are not gouged by providers. This may in turn lead to a stiffening of the resolve of certain employers who want to back up their employees with regard to interaction with the health system. But don't hold your breath.

The key trend for employers will be to find a way to build viable managed care models that suit an emerging workforce that is looking to be more flexible, more fluid, more adaptable, and more likely to move from one employer to another on short notice. The health benefit structure for the present seems to be somewhat archaic, and there is an opportunity for health insurers to design products and services that are more tailored to the needs of the new economy. We need products that are portable, expandable, contractable, and tailored to different budgets and needs.

Similarly, policymakers have to look long and hard at the viability of employment-based health insurance as the anchor for coverage in the future. Surveys indicate bipartisan satisfaction with health insurance; "If it ain't broke, don't fix it" seems to be the mantra. However, the rising number of uninsured is testimony that the employment-based health insurance market is not thriving but, on the contrary, is offering poor value, at least as perceived by many employers and their employees.

Harris surveys indicate that employers have been generally satisfied over the last ten years as their burden of health costs has slowed and as they've transferred more of the obligation on to consumers. Going forward, one can imagine that employers will still be relatively happy as they insulate themselves from double-digit premium increases by transferring the burden onto consumers. Therefore, don't expect employers to lead the charge for wholesale health reform. They will not be leaders in the future the way they were leaders in promoting the more rapid penetration of managed care during the last recession. If a revolution is to come, it is more likely to come out of the discontent of consumers. We turn now to their plight.

Chapter Eight

Consumers

We've Seen the Enemy and It's Helen Hunt

Consumers want what they can't have. Like Helen Hunt's character in the movie *As Good As It Gets,* the average consumer wants to spend an unbelievable amount of time talking to high-paid medical professionals who listen to their every concern about their life and about their health problems. Then, if these caring professionals identify any potential disease, they conduct an enormous battery of tests on the patient's behalf, and the patient pays nothing for it.

In large measure, this scenario is the idealized fee-for-service system of the past—the good old days remembered by doctors. At least it was the good old days when the patient was armed with third-party indemnity insurance and when the physicians, not stressed by managed care, were able to set prices that would allow them to spend half an hour with each patient and still generate their target income. Those good old days have been severely altered by the increasing complexity of medicine, by the intensity of demands on physicians' time brought about by managed care, and by the perceived constraint on physicians' target incomes. Consumers, rather than being less demanding as a result of managed care, are more demanding. Consumers want more for less, as in most other fields.

New Consumers Call the Shots

What is behind this rising consumerism and the in-your-face nature of consumer interaction with physicians? Clearly one of the primary driving forces is the aging of the baby boomers and the generations that follow them. Half of the baby boom went to college. Half of that half made it through college, and among the cohorts that follow, 60 to 70 percent have had at least one year of college education. As noted in Chapter Three, those who have had at least one year of college tend to behave similarly to those who have college degrees, so these individuals are somewhat undifferentiated from college graduates in their sophistication and demanding nature. In the book *The Second Curve,* I talked about the role of new consumers and how they are likely to change the health system. In particular, I argued that the true Second Curve of health care would involve the health care system using new technology (particularly the Internet) to interact with better-informed, skeptical, and demanding consumers in new ways, for example by providing e-commerce connections between patients and doctors.

Emerging Consumer Segments

Undeniably, there are new consumers in the marketplace. A large proportion of the U.S. public has college education and access to the Internet. They are skeptical and demanding in all that they do. They make lousy employees. They are terribly difficult customers. They demand high quality and low cost, and they're not willing to pay much out of pocket for services. Essentially, the Internet generation expects everything to be free. So meeting the demands of consumers is becoming increasingly hard. But it would be wrong to assume that all consumers fall into that skeptical, demanding, willing-to-trade-up-with-their-own-money segment. Indeed, careful analysis by Louis Harris and the Harvard School of Public Health in a recent Strategic Health Perspectives study found that there were three clearly identifiable emerging groups in the consumer market.

The first group is the *trade-up players,* amounting to some 9 percent of the American public. These individuals, who tend to have higher income and education, have, will, and can pay more for treatments and provider choice. They actively seek information about their health; for example, 49 percent have looked for information about a health topic on-line compared to 27 percent of the total population.

A second, much larger group, accounting for 23 percent of the population, is made up of the *reluctantly empowered*. These are people who have paid more for care but are not willing to do so regularly. They have had to make choices involuntarily to get back to the open-ended health benefits they once enjoyed. For a variety of reasons, including changes in their health benefits and shifts from defined-benefit to defined-contribution plans, these consumers are being forced to pay more out of pocket for their health costs.

The third group is the *needy shoppers*, primarily those on Medicaid and the uninsured, some 23 percent of the population. People in this group will pay for services they perceive they want or need and don't have, even if they can't afford it. This group, despite lower income and inadequate coverage, exhibits consumerist behaviors but is doing so to get its just due in the health care system. In particular, Medicaid recipients exhibit a higher interest in improved customer service and amenities such as waiting rooms, and more willingness to pay for it, than almost any other group. This interest in service factors reflects the baseline from which they are responding to this question. In particular, the level of customer service among safety-net providers is not particularly sophisticated. Needy shoppers, however meager their resources, indicate they're willing to pay out of pocket to get more appropriate treatment and better customer service.

In total, these three segments still account for only a little more than half of all consumers of U.S. health care. Humphrey Taylor, chairman of Louis Harris and Associates, has described the remainder as the primordial stew of consumer segmentation. The metaphor is appropriate. If one thinks about it for a second, it seems silly to suggest that all consumers are in clearly defined segments in health care, because in the past health has not been a consumer good. It has not been paid for directly by the consumer. Indeed there is a thirty- to forty-year trend of consumers paying directly an ever smaller share of the health care dollar. It is only in the last two to three years that this trend has turned around to any degree. And that turnaround is minor compared to the long-run trend of insulating the consumer from the cost of health care. So one would not really expect consumerist behavior the way one sees it in relation to packaged goods, entertainment, or consumer goods such as stereo equipment or automobiles.

Changes in Consumer Behavior

As consumers are pushed into a position of being the payers for more of the health care dollar, they are likely to select among options very different from those offered in the past. For example, alternative medicine is going to become a major staple for a more aggressive, assertive baby boomer who appreciates some of the New Age values or spiritual or broader holistic healing methods embodied in alternative and complementary medicine approaches— regardless of whether or not the science is behind them.

A second key area where we are going to see consumers make major changes is in the entire informational infrastructure for health care. The Internet clearly is going to be a driving force and a platform for allowing pluralism to reign among consumer preferences with regard to gathering health information. As we have seen, sixty million Americans went on-line for health information in 1998 alone. But health on the Net is still an immature industry. The plethora of Web sites offering health information range from those giving serious scientifically based information to flaky Web sites spawned by some kid in a basement. Jennifer Wayne Doppke, an expert on Internet usage in health care, has likened health care on the Internet to cable TV: 10 percent is *Masterpiece Theatre* and 90 percent is Jerry Springer.

The Internet, then, is going to be a significant vehicle for enabling consumers not only to be diverse in their informational experiences but also to build communities of interest among members of disease groups and among those who share particular concerns. E-commerce on the Web will also be a vehicle for health plans, provider groups, and others to keep in touch with their patients and deliver services as well as provide the backbone for the administration of health care in the future.

A third key area of impact of the more activist consumers will be in their role as voters. This is an important part of the future landscape because consumers behave simultaneously as patients, as enrollees in health plans, and as voters. More than 10 percent of Americans are also employed in the health care system, with another 5 to 10 percent dependent on business from the health care industry.

Consumers as Voters

It is the consumer as voter who can have the most major impact on health care. As a greater burden is placed on consumers to pay for care, they are going to become more activist in political terms. The long-running Harris survey on consumer satisfaction in health care shows that the proportion who think the system works pretty well and only needs minor changes has begun to fall again. At the other extreme, the proportion of Americans believing that the health care system has a great deal wrong with it and needs to be completely rebuilt is increasing. Although the level of discontent has not reached the historic highs of the pre-Clinton health plan era of 1994, there are clear signs that dissatisfaction is beginning to increase again.

Public dissatisfaction with health care has both cyclical and long-term structural components. Dissatisfaction is linked to the business cycle, and therefore if we were to dip into recession, the number of discontented Americans would rise significantly. But dissatisfaction also has structural dimensions; a steady erosion of public confidence in health care is a long-term trend. If public discontent rises to a threshold at which health care becomes *the* top political issue, there will be another major health care reform debate. We are not there yet.

The key health policy priorities for the next decade will likely be in reforming Medicare and making incremental improvements in coverage. First, modernizing Medicare and preserving the safety net for seniors, along with Social Security, is the top health and social policy agenda item. The aging of the baby boom and its effect on Medicare and Social Security will be the most salient political driver over the next twenty years.

Second, incremental expansion of coverage is a likely goal that can take many forms. Expansion for the near-elderly or maturing baby boomers of fifty-five to sixty-four, allowing them to buy into Medicare, has already been proposed. This is a politically astute proposition because of the higher voting prevalence in the older age groups and because health care is an issue of more salience for an aging population.

Little or no attention has been given to broader expansion for the uninsured, albeit that the Kiddie Care legislation was passed in 1997 to provide some support and to reduce the number of uninsured children. But there is no policy move toward expanding coverage to the young adult population who comprise the vast majority of the uninsured.

Consumer protection issues became politically popular in the late 1990s as the legislative manifestation of the consumer backlash. Regulation of managed care is politically appealing because it doesn't appear to cost anything. Perversely, however, by protecting consumers from the ravages of managed care we may in some senses be aggravating the uninsured problem because of regulatory restrictions on managed care plans, particularly those requiring that patients have access to specialists. These regulations may price managed care out of the market even further as premiums rise and as managed care becomes defanged in the name of quality, which will only further aggravate the coverage issue.

Resolving the tensions between regulating managed care and expanding affordable coverage, between preserving and modernizing Medicare simultaneously, and between adding to Medicare benefits and containing costs may be too much to ask of our political leaders. These are inherently conflicting policy goals. There is a natural political tendency to promise more than can be delivered.

Consumers, Technology, and Rationing

Consumers may be directly confronted with the very difficult question that we as a society collectively need to face: Will we provide all of the fruits of medical technology to every single one of our citizens, to provide even the smallest of improvement in health benefit? New medical technology is likely to continue to be both expensive and effective. However, the degree to which we make these technologies available to all will depend on our willingness to pay for them. So far the American public has been reluctant to be drawn into a rationing debate. Rationing is not an American value. The Oregon Medicaid experiment was an attempt at rationing in which policymakers, health professionals, and lay advisory groups drawn from the community rank-ordered Medicaid procedures according to their perceived cost-effectiveness and impact on health. By refusing to pay for cosmetic surgery for example, Medicaid could cover well-baby visits. This pioneering model for the nation has struggled. If it doesn't sell in Oregon, it will have an even tougher job in other states, such as New York. Bear in mind that Oregon has relatively low health care costs, does not have very generous Medicaid benefits, and has a very low population of minorities. (This last characteristic has a significant impact on the politics of rationing for Medicaid recipients.)

The rationing debate has not gained any currency in the national forum, and politicians are unlikely to touch it. Managed care, as we have seen, has been suckered into being the default rationer in U.S. health care, and it has been demonized as a result. Given the power of technology, its likely costs, and the continued demands of the public for state of the art, Helen Hunt will have to be brought into the debate about limits on expenditure and limits on service. This need for consumer participation is particularly important when it comes to debate about services in the last years of life. Although it is popular for many pundits to say that 30 percent of health care costs are consumed in the last year of life, this is really an overstatement. The data indicate that a third of *Medicare* costs occur in the last year of life. Medicare is only about a third of all health care costs. The vast majority of health care costs are not incurred in the last year of life, although it is true that an ever increasing proportion is consumed in the final years of life.

Victor Fuchs, a noted health economist at Stanford University, points to the trends in utilization for the older-age cohorts. The following are some examples of the average annual rate of increase in use of certain procedures per 100,000 elderly in the eighty-five-year-old and older range, from 1987 to 1995: 22 percent for angioplasty, 15 percent for coronary artery bypass surgery, 16 percent for cardiac cauterization, 11 percent for carotid endarterectomy, 26 percent for hip replacement, 11 percent for knee replacement, and 8 percent for laminectomy. This rapid increase in utilization of services is taking place in the population currently over eighty-five—and this is a generation that knows the meaning of sacrifice. Less than 10 percent have college education; they grew up struggling through the 1930s; many of them served in World War II. This is a generation that has sacrificed, yet we are seeing enormous increases in utilization—clearly a harbinger of significant future rates of growth in technologies to alleviate pain and suffering and improve quality of life in the very old. Imagine what it will be like when we have a bunch of cranky eighty-five-year-old baby boomers who have always expected the world to be handed to them on a plate. We boomers are all going to be sitting around in nursing homes singing "I've Got You Babe" to each other, demanding Viagra, clamoring for total hip replacements so we can continue to play tennis and golf, and insisting on frequent renewal of our cardiovascular plumbing systems to enable us to be active and to travel and enjoy the world.

Walter Bortz, a leading gerontologist at Stanford University and the Palo Alto Medical Clinic, advocates a more holistic view of health and promotes the understanding that with appropriate lifestyle and dietary changes, there is no reason why significant proportions of the population can't live to be one hundred. Indeed, centenarians are the fasting-growing cohort in the U.S. population; there are projected to be more than 65,000 people over one hundred years old by the year 2000.

How we will live in our older age will be one of the central political and economic questions of the next decade. The public policy debate will involve Social Security and Medicare, to be sure, but it will also involve discussion about a more holistic view of health and well-being in retirement and about long-term care, housing, and transportation. The aging of America really begins in the twenty-first century, and the rapid escalation in the proportion of the population over sixty-five occurs in 2010 and beyond. American society will be completely transformed by an elderly baby boom, just as it was when the baby boom entered schools, colleges, and the workplace. And don't underestimate the role that information technology will play among this new group of seniors in the delivery of health services and social support.

Helen Hunt in the Future

Overall, Helen Hunt is aging gracefully. But she is demanding more from the health system even though she is struggling to make ends meet and provide health insurance for her family. Helen Hunt's predicament is likely to get worse before it gets better. The typical single mother who is marginally employed in the restaurant trade is unlikely to get better health insurance benefits over the next decade; in fact she is likely to get worse benefits. It is true that if her income is low enough, her children will have access to health insurance through the Kiddie Care program, provided the state in which she lives (in this case New York) is capable of organizing a system to reach out and enroll her child. For her own health insurance, she will have to depend on the luck of coming across a wealthy customer who, though quirky, would be kind enough to provide access to specialists for her. If she expects that kind of service to continue in the future, then some fundamental changes in the nature of coverage for working people will have to be undertaken.

As Helen ages, the questions about linking health coverage to employment become more troubling. It's not inconceivable that in her late fifties she will find waitressing too much for her; will she be able to find a job with health insurance? Will she be allowed to buy into Medicare? These are troubling issues for an aging baby boom.

As we look further out, will Helen be able to have access to all of the medical technologies available to future physicians? Will she have exactly the same kind of coverage as other kinds of Medicare recipients in 2020? Will Medicare be a universal program for all? Will it even cover all elderly? How old will Helen have to be to qualify? Will managed care help her access affordable health care, or will it continue to frustrate her? These are all questions that Helen Hunt can not only look forward to but also actually help shape in her role as a voter and as a U.S. citizen.

Chapter Nine

After the Backlash

Strategies for Survival of Managed Care

For twenty years, managed care has been the answer to the American health care crisis. Now we seem to have put this particular ship into a fairly steep reverse. However, it is important neither to abandon all that has been gained in managed care nor to suggest that we have another good idea beyond managed care. The simple fact is that Americans don't do government. Most other countries use government as the primary source of funding and use top-down restraint on public funding as the primary lever for containing costs. Despite moves toward privatization, most countries—including Canada, the United Kingdom, Sweden, and Germany—still effectively contain costs through global budgets. In the United States, managed care is all we've got to build on as a mechanism for reconciling cost, quality, and access.

Managed Care and Managed Care Lite

The core model of managed care, the group and staff model HMO—Kaiser Permanente, Harvard Pilgrim Health Care, Group Health of Puget Sound, and the Henry Ford Health System of Detroit being prime examples—has come under significant criticism for being sluggish and unresponsive to the communities these plans serve. Critics anticipated that the newer managed care organizations would be more nimble, more flexible, and more virtually

135

integrated, using information technology and contracts to link together a diverse provider network. The consumer-friendly, virtually integrated, indemnity-like health insurance plans—managed care lite—were somehow to provide a more market-oriented, responsive, and flexible architecture for the delivery of health services. However, these plans too have struggled.

The Old Hard Core of Managed Care

It is wrong to assume that the organizations of the past have nothing to offer in the future. Kaiser, Henry Ford, and Harvard Pilgrim in particular are important organizations to monitor for the future because of their contributions in the past, their infrastructure, and their missions to improve quality, contain costs, and reform the medical care system. Kaiser Permanente is trying to prove a point rather than simply make money. And the point is that medicine can be organized, that systems of care can be coordinated, that investment in organization can yield systematic improvement in the way in which patients are managed, and that all this can be combined with compassion and high quality of physician-patient relationships. Coordination of care, integration of services, and compassion for the community have been the hallmarks of these organizations in the past.

Kaiser, Henry Ford, Harvard Pilgrim and similar organizations were given the green light by the theory of managed competition, which was predicated on the idea of competition for informed cost-conscious consumers among large, vertically integrated actors. However, it is unlikely that all segments of the American public are going to accept or desire to be involved in such vertically integrated systems. Kaiser and other vertically integrated plans are recognizing that they must carve a dominant position in the segments to which they are most attractive, namely working Americans and retirees on Medicare who value coordinated care.

Aside from the high-quality service provided to working people, these large, not-for-profit HMOs are the only organizations that are making investments of the scale required to transform medical practice. If there is a central challenge going forward for the managed care industry as a whole, it is in making medical management a reality, in finding ways in which medical management can be done successfully. Doing so requires that plans make an investment in infrastructure—both information systems and intellectual capital—to innovate in the care delivery system and to manage medical care more effectively. Kaiser and the other large-scale integrated systems have made significant investments in this area. For example, Kaiser Permanente Medical Group of Northern California held an innovations conference in 1994 in San Francisco. Moscone Center was full of Kaiser employees from Northern California, complete with booths just like a trade show, except that the only participants were Kaiser employees. The conference celebrated innovations in clinical practice, in management technology, in coordination of care, and in improvement of quality. Few for-profit managed care plans make this kind of research investment in care delivery or in such intellectual apparatus for improving medical management.

But, like much of managed care, these integrated systems have struggled and perhaps faired worse than some of their for-profit competitors in the late 1990s. Overall, group and staff model HMOs stopped growing in 1990, although Kaiser and some others have regained members and market share in certain metropolitan areas. Some analysts have argued that the pursuit of growth has severely affected these organizations' bottom line and that they might have been better trying to preserve rather than grow market share.

Managed Care Lite

In terms of market share, the winners in managed care in the late 1980s and early 1990s have clearly been those in the lite model of managed care. Managed care lite is predicated on four basic instruments. The first of these is selective contracting with providers. Rather than build anything, one can simply contract with physicians. And there's no limit to the number of managed care plans that can enter a market because physicians have shown an amazing ability to contract with multiple organizations. Initially, typical U.S. physicians liked this model because it essentially fulfilled their goal of making sure that no one payer had control over their business. The lite managed care players then can selectively contract among doctors, and the typical physician has anywhere from five to twenty different managed care contracts and will in addition accept almost any form of third-party coverage on a full-indemnity basis.

The second instrument of managed care lite is some form of utilization review, ranging all the way from preadmission certification for hospital stays, to specialty referral controls, to the use of gatekeeper physicians. This latter innovation has proved increasingly unpopular with the U.S. public, however. Indeed, as discussed in Chapter Five, restrictions on specialty referrals have been a major stimulus of the demonization of managed care, because unfettered access to specialists in the United States is the surrogate for quality. Much of the utilization control in the world of lite managed care is predicated on nifty claims analysis. Bear in mind that a medical claim is a creative fiction in which the provider and the patient conspire against the third-party insurance company. Basing medical management on claims analysis is a little bit like steering an airplane by looking at the passenger manifest: there's little or no connection.

It is interesting to look at Canada, where primary care physicians act as the gatekeepers do in the U.S. managed care environment. In Canada, patients can go directly to specialists. There is no restriction on them making appointments directly, but most specialists will not accept an appointment with a patient directly without a referral from a general practitioner; if they do, they get reimbursed for a primary care visit. In other words, the health plan (in this case the government) places incentives on the physician to refer appropriately, rather than making it apparent to the patient that he or she has been denied access to specialty referral by the health plan. It's a subtle difference, but one that I think would be interesting to try in the U.S. context. Indeed, the Blue Shield of California Access Plus HMO is really a U.S. version of this model. Patients are asked to pay for the specialty referral (or a significant proportion of it) through a higher copayment when they self-refer to a specialist without going through their gatekeeper physician.

The third instrument of managed care lite is the financial incentives to both patient and physician. A number of different financial incentives can be used, including risk pools, withholds, and capitation. For example, in the delegated, capitated model, a medical group is given capitation payments, either to cover its services, to cover its services and ancillary services, or to cover all physician services. In some cases, depending on state licensing and regulation, large-scale medical groups can receive full (or total) capitation to cover all physician services and all hospital services. The capitation model grew rapidly in the late 1980s and early 1990s but has stalled to some degree in the late 1990s because of a lack of medical groups with the sophistication to manage capitation.

The more prevalent model for reimbursement is for IPAs and other networks to accept either a capitated contract or a discounted fee for service with some withholding that is at risk depending on the IPAs' performance in terms of total cost and quality. This model allows groups to absorb some of the risk and reward for reducing utilization.

Similarly, lite plans (such as traditional indemnity health insurance) provide incentives for patients in the form of user fees—copays and deductibles and tiering of those copays and deductibles to keep those patients within a certain network of providers. There is an enormous international literature on user fees that refutes the American premise that consumers paying user fees out of pocket somehow control overall health costs. Most Canadian and British health economists would regard that assertion as patent nonsense. Canadian and non-U.S. economists argue that because of the concentration of health care costs in a very small number of people who have serious diseases, charging these people user fees is unlikely to control total costs. Also, it is a false economy to prevent people from accessing primary care through the use of user fees that may encourage them to postpone treatment and end up requiring more significant treatment down the line.

It is true that one can steer patients around a health system by using copays and deductibles, the POS plan being a good example. Another good example is tiered formularies for prescription drugs; consumers are asked now to pay anywhere from $5 to $40 of copayment, depending on the cost of their medication. This trend will increase in the future.

No matter how offensive user fees may be to those around the world who believe it is a false economy, it is an inherently American solution. Cost sharing by the consumer addresses a common American concern, namely that because the patient doesn't pay the full costs of care, there is a greater likelihood of inappropriate escalation in utilization.

The final instrument of managed care lite, and a fundamental principle of the HMO movement from the beginning, has been the emphasis on wellness and prevention. Here the progress has been mixed. Although the U.S. public sees a great deal of value in prevention, HMOs have not really given people much in the way of prevention. To be fair, compared to traditional fee-for-service models, HMOs have been much more likely to include coverage for well-baby visits, for prenatal care, for screening tests, and for annual physicals. It is also the case that many of the capitated medical groups went so far as doing interventions in the homes of elderly patients to prevent accidents and falls so as to avoid the large medical costs associated with the result of such events (such as total hip replacement).

Although managed care has demonstrated greater focus on wellness and prevention than have fee-for-service models, it is still true that prevention or, more broadly, the systematic attention to the determinants of health have not really been the focus of most HMOs. For example, HMOs have not been aggressively antismoking, and there have been little or no major improvements or actions by HMOs with regard to such issues as violence or traffic safety. So in terms of taking a broader view of health, HMOs have tended to be focused more on management of sick care and on avoiding payment for sick care, rather than on really stimulating prevention and wellness in a much broader, holistic way.

These four instruments of managed care lite—selective contracting, utilization review and medical management, financial incentives, and wellness and prevention—have been reasonably successful to date in mirroring the broad performance characteristics of a vertically integrated HMO such as Kaiser. Using these four instruments, managed care lite has ameliorated the increase in health costs while meeting two important objectives: first, providing patients with choice to navigate their way around the health system among independent physicians, and second, not requiring that individual physicians put all their eggs in one organizational basket by either joining a large group or becoming an employee or signing an exclusive contract with one managed care health plan. Pluralism has been served.

The degree of coordination and the investment by lite managed care in medical management technology have not been nearly as great as in the not-for-profit plans. There are some exceptions to this generalization, however. United HealthCare has an affiliated company originally called Applied Health Informatics, now a separate company called Ingenix. Ingenix has over four hundred employees, many of whom are serious health policy researchers and medical statisticians, who have carefully mined United HealthCare's data sets to identify best practices, not only for United HealthCare but also for the other clients they serve. Increasingly Ingenix will be an independent voice and an independent player in producing practice guidelines and best practices for use by other managed care organizations. But Ingenix is unusual. Few of the other for-profit HMOs have the same kind of research function dedicated to improving the performance of managed care.

The challenge for managed care lite going forward is to identify ways in which to encourage medical management and to maintain and improve quality without necessarily having to integrate physician practices physically, organizationally, and culturally. Virtual integration, Web-enabled interaction—these are positive and consistent with the American notion of pluralism. But many believe, and a good deal of the evidence suggests, that it is only when providers practice "shoulder to shoulder medicine" and when the cultural controls of peers managing peers really are brought to bear that significant changes in behavior can occur. Many in the lite managed care world refute this notion and suggest that there is as much, if not more, potential for dramatic improvements in utilization through the use of technology to coordinate the activities of far-flung independent physicians and to make them behave as if they were following one culture. Ingenix is pursuing that strategy on behalf of United and its other HMO clients. It remains to be seen whether we can build the infrastructure to make this vision of managed care lite a reality. For now, the industry seems to be struggling to find a way to navigate its way to this new medical management nirvana.

Strategic Menu for Health Plans

All organizations, whether they are for-profit or nonprofit, have to be concerned about growth, about margin, and about sustainable, defensible positions. For-profit plans have to deliver growth and earnings per share and continued profitability to their Wall Street investors and have to demonstrate to the shareholders that they are worth hanging onto for the long run because of a sustainable, defensible strategy. But similarly, Kaiser and the other large not-for-profit plans have bondholders who are interested in the financial, long-term viability of these plans. Not-for-profit doesn't mean that you don't make profit; it means that the program is of sufficient social value that the status of not paying taxes is granted to the organization.

The following sections describe several strategies for growth, several strategies for margin, and strategies for defense that all health plans must consider.

Adding New Lives

A managed care plan can add new lives by capturing market share from competitors or by going after public sector managed care lives in Medicare and Medicaid.

Medicare

Up until 1998, Medicare was one of the key sources of growth in managed care enrollment through the Medicare risk program (now called Medicare+Choice). In essence the program allowed health plans to recruit seniors into HMOs provided they were offered a benefit package at least as good as Medicare. The plan would be paid 95 percent of the prevailing costs for a Medicare recipient in that county—the average adjusted per capita cost (AAPCC) rate, established by the HCFA for each county in the United States as a per capita monthly payment to an HMO on behalf of a Medicare beneficiary.

PacifiCare is the leader in the Medicare risk business, with over a third of all Medicare lives nationally enrolled through its Secure Horizons brand health plan. Overall, PacifiCare was one of the leading lights of managed care from the mid-1980s to the mid-

1990s. PacifiCare faltered somewhat after the acquisition of competitor FHP and as Medicare became less profitable as a business line in the late 1990s.

The key challenge in Medicare risk is that it requires enrolling the elderly one life at a time, unlike large-group benefits for which hundreds or thousands of employees can be signed up by one salesperson. Industry statistics indicate that it costs approximately $1,000 per life to market and establish a health plan for Medicare recipients. Similarly, experts in the field regard thirty thousand lives per market as the minimum number required to have a sustainable HMO position. Alternatively, HMOs can reach the same size threshold through a combination of commercial and Medicare lives—one hundred thousand commercial lives being the break-even point (a Medicare life in premium terms being three to four times a commercial life).

A setup target of $1,000 per life requires a $30 million investment one way or another in any new market that an HMO chooses to enter. Such heavy start-up marketing costs are one reason that provider-sponsored network (PSN) Medicare plans have been unattractive. (A PSN plan is an HMO owned and run by hospitals or doctors.) Why would you pay $30 million in marketing costs so you can decrease your overall utilization of your own hospitals? It makes no sense for a PSN to get into that business except in extreme cases as a defensive strategy, but even then it's sort of turning on yourself.

HMOs have been successful in Medicare risk when the AAPCC rate is high, where there is high awareness of managed care but little competition for Medicare business, and where there is a group of appropriate providers (GPs and specialists) willing and sophisticated enough to accept capitation. It also helps if the markets have huge numbers of specialists, high utilization of hospitals, and savvy elderly consumers.

In the early days there were real easy pickings. One could go to Miami or Los Angeles and reduce hospital utilization significantly (as measured by bed days per thousand population) and reap an enormous bounty, particularly if one could identify healthier lives to enroll in the first place. Medicare HMOs reaped significant rewards, as did the capitated providers who were there at the early stage. But like pyramid schemes, purchasing of Yahoo! or amazon.com stock, Ponzi schemes, and chain letters, the riches go to the early adopters, and when these bubbles eventually burst, the average punter is left holding the bag.

Medicare+Choice could still be an important platform for future health reform. But if it is to work in the long run, there must be enough incentive for the managed care plans to maintain their presence in the Medicare+Choice market. That will require rate adjustments over time so that these Medicare HMOs can earn a reasonable rate of return. However, as Uwe Reinhardt, a Princeton health economist, has pointed out, it is likely that the Medicare HMO of the future is going to look a lot more like a regulated electric utility than an independent free enterprise organization. (It is somewhat ironic that the electric power industry is sort of passing the health industry as they go in opposite directions: just as we are regulating HMOs to look more like electric utilities, so electric utilities are deregulating to look more like managed care. In the deregulated environment, electric utilities are no longer granted monopolies on an end-to-end basis to generate, distribute, and market electric power. Rather, with utility reform the various parts of the generation, distribution, and marketing of electricity will be parsed out, and there will be competition among the various actors, analogous to the vision of managed care and managed competition of the early 1980s and through the 1990s.)

Medicare+Choice, as we have seen, is a central opportunity for the managed care industry to go forward, but being in bed with the federal government as your long-term business partner is a tricky proposition. The relationships between the HCFA and the managed care industry have not been nearly as cozy as the ones between the Pentagon and the defense industry over the years. There are few HCFA players in the managed care industry, and vice versa. So over time, better relationships between these organizations need to be fostered. However, it is fair to say that the HCFA has always looked to PacifiCare's Secure Horizons Medicare HMO as the paragon of private sector Medicare managed care.

Medicaid

Medicaid represents a significant opportunity in terms of enrollment of new members, but the real question mark with Medicaid HMOs, at least for for-profit, private alliances, is whether they can be money makers, given the low level of funding per capita in the Medicaid program. The short answer is probably yes if one looks at AFDC lite—in other words, at those enrollees in the AFDC program who do not have comorbidities, typically young healthy mothers and kids. The private sector is much less interested in signing up on a capitated-risk basis those patients who need long-term care or care under the Medicaid program to the disabled. It is unlikely that significant, viable, for-profit arrangements can be easily orchestrated in those areas, especially if doing so involves rationing for the blind, the disabled, or the elderly. Consequently, for-profit Medicaid HMOs are likely to have a rocky road, and the only people likely to be aggressive in the pursuit of this strategy will be those who can add Medicaid to other lines of business to provide further consolidation (for example, WellPoint or Foundation Health, both of which have Medi-Cal HMOs in California).

New Aggregators

Aggregators are businesses, associations, or cooperatives that bring together lives to be covered by insurance. New aggregators offer potential new channels of distribution for insurance product, and there are some exciting new channels being developed. Automated Data Processing (ADP) processes much of the payroll for small and medium-size business in America. They recently purchased Health Benefits of America (HBA), which is in the business of outsourcing managed care administration services. This business provides large employers, such as Marriott, with private-label HMO capacity by contracting with the HMOs and providing all the benefit enrollment and administrative services necessary to do open enrollment and manage the managed care entities for large employers. HBA has been very successful in this field, and ADP brings the kind of marketing, reach, and clout to extend those services to a much wider population, including the growing number of medium-size companies.

Professional employee organizations (PEOs), known sometimes as employee leasing companies, provide a new form of aggregation of employees. Similarly, there is the potential for creation of new health purchasing cooperatives by employer groups, such as the Pacific Business Group on Health (who recently took over the management of the California state health insurance purchasing cooperative [HIPC] for small businesses), or other organizations put together by benefit consultants, such as Towers-Perrin or Hewitt and Associates.

Becoming an Acquisition Machine

Horizontal consolidation through acquisition is a key growth mechanism accepted by Wall Street. Aggressive consolidators can roll up business entities and keep growth rates and their earnings per share positive by using their stock as currency. In the managed care industry, consolidation seems to be one of the key default strategies for the future. It is much easier to acquire than to build through organic growth. Organic growth, as we have seen, requires significant investment in marketing. In a fiercely competitive commercial insurance market, costs can run as high as $1,000 per life, almost exactly that for a Medicare life, and therefore going after market growth on an organic basis requires a significant outlay of capital. It is much less expensive to acquire lives through acquisition provided that Wall Street cooperates by rewarding acquisitions with higher stock prices. The consolidators in the business—WellPoint, United, Cigna, and Aetna U.S. Healthcare—have been rewarded. Multiline insurers, such as Cigna and Aetna, can also use profits from other lines of business to purchase at the bottom of the cycle for managed care, and they have consistently done so. On the upturns in the cycle, these companies generate large profits, which in turn can dampen the cycles of their other businesses, provided that their line of businesses are not all tanking at the same time.

A variant on the consolidation strategy popular in the early 1990s was conversion from lite to heavy managed care. In 1994, indemnity and PPO lives could be purchased for between $80 to $200 per life; if blocks of such lives could be converted to HMO status, they would be valued by Wall Street at $1,000 to $4,000 per life. This strategy was really the core of the Metra Health strategy. Metropolitan Life and Travelers had a significant number of lite managed care lives, which they folded together in a joint venture called Metra. Metra struggled to add any value to the managed care business largely because it was still an indemnity-focused business. United HealthCare then bought those lives for less than $200 a life. Had they been able to convert them directly to HMO lives overnight, they would have significantly raised the value of their stock; to some degree this did occur, and United was successful in growing its core HMO business using these lighter lives as a feeding ground. But in another sense, it was less easy than United and others thought in making that conversion, because a PPO is a different product line; it's a different selling proposition with different product features that appeal to a different constituency. Just because a customer signs up for a PPO doesn't mean that he or she is going to take your HMO. So crossing the bridge from PPO to HMO has not been as easy as some might have thought.

Annexing the Sudetenland

A third growth strategy is what I call "annexing the Sudetenland" (named after one unpopular acquirer's strategic method). The notion here is that an HMO can migrate to another geography, particularly from the advanced managed care markets, such as California, to less advanced markets. The strategy seems plausible enough but has met with mixed success. In its migration to Georgia, WellPoint has demonstrated an ability to go after other markets. Foundation Health Systems has had difficulty in going outside of its core marketplaces to such places as Philadelphia. PacifiCare also has had mixed results outside of its core markets in the West; even with its Medicare managed care expertise, PacifiCare struggled in Florida.

Part of the problem for those plans that have gone outside California with the intention of using capitation and delegation as a strategy (PacifiCare being the most notable example) is a lack of physician leaders with managed care savvy in the community they enter. It is what I have termed the "Where is Bob Margolis?" problem. Dr. Robert Margolis is a prominent Los Angeles leader in the world of large group practices and has been a loyal and important member of the PacifiCare network. Margolis's Health Partners Group is the largest independent capitated group practice left standing in Southern California; it was not swept into the Med-Partners–Mullikin consolidation (the publicly traded large group practice company) and has remained relatively independent. Margolis's organization has remained diligently focused on primary care–based models of managing care for both commercially insured HMO patients and Medicare managed care patients. Health Partners has been one of the key network building blocks for those plans, such as Health Net, PacifiCare, and WellPoint, that valued and exploited the capitated, delegated model. So when these plans move out of California, they obviously like to find somebody like Bob Margolis in their new markets. So where's Waldo? It's not as easy as you might think to spot the Bob Margolis in a crowd of doctors. It becomes a very significant challenge, and indeed in many parts of the country such physicians and such group practices simply don't exist.

In 1994, the Institute for the Future conducted a study of these integrated health systems and large group practices; the researchers came to the conclusion that the single most important core competency behind these successfully capitated and integrated groups was that they had been doing it for twenty years! By definition, this is a very difficult core competency to re-create overnight, and indeed one of the key factors underlying the lack of more rapid diffusion in capitation is really the absence of physician leaders like Bob Margolis.

Another key impediment in trying to move out of the California model was the assumption made by many California managed care players that reducing the overutilization on the East Coast was going to be easy pickings—low-hanging fruit they could easily exploit. For example, at its height, the hospitalization utilization under Oxford Health Plan's Medicare risk contract was 2,400 days per thousand, whereas in Southern California at the same time some of the medical groups were running as low as 800 to 1,100 days per thousand. California plans looked at these New York numbers and said, "Boy, there's lots of money to be made out there." However, the prevailing days per thousand in the New York market were up around 3,600 or 4,200—way above the national average of 2,400. At its height, Oxford succeeded only in getting utilization levels in New York to the national average. Part of the reason for that discrepancy is the nature of medical practice in the New York marketplace: it is much more hospital intensive. Californians got carried away with the days-per-thousand mantra in the 1990s, thinking that by reducing days per thousand they were also reducing cost, and this really is a California fallacy.

As Dr. Stuart Altman, a health economist at Brandeis University, has observed, nobody actually ever goes to a hospital in California. Indeed, what we've done in California is turn people's living rooms into ICUs. The California model has been to move care to so-called less expensive settings, although this points to the fallacy that by moving the hospital care into a home or ambulatory environment, it necessarily becomes less expensive. Uwe Reinhardt of Princeton University has pointed out that Americans don't know how to do cost accounting, and as a consequence they imagine that the average cost of care is actually equivalent to the marginal cost of care, which is a glaring error from both an accounting and an economic standpoint. In other words, assuming that the cost of a day in the hospital is $1,000 may be totally accurate for the first two or three days of stay. It is not accurate for the tenth day of stay, because a hospital really is a Holiday Inn with gasses. Most of the marginal costs of care are not much greater than hotel costs. It is what we choose to do to patients in hospitals that makes hospitals expensive—the equipment and so forth that is wheeled into their rooms for particular sets of events. Thus, cutting stays down by a day doesn't necessarily mean you're going to reduce costs by that proportion of the stay, because length of stay and cost are not necessarily correlated. The intervening variable is intensity of servicing.

This difference between marginal costs and average costs explains why Canadian hospitals are less expensive. Canada's length of stay is longer, but intensity of servicing per day is much less. Britain and Japan are even more extreme; patients stay a long time in hospitals but with very low intensity of service per day. Japan, indeed, has the longest lengths of stay in the world but one of the lowest hospital costs per capita among developed countries. In the California case, intensity of servicing during the remaining hospital stays is extremely high and remains extremely high even under managed care.

So the fallacy of regional migration of managed care was that the kinds of days per thousand that existed in California could be applied in the New York or Boston market and that a proportional reduction in those lengths of stay would yield enormous profits. That has not proven to be the case; although a significant reduction in lengths of stay and utilization of hospitals has been achieved, it is not to the level of the California numbers, nor, as we have just discussed, would that level necessarily be equivalent to a significant cost reduction.

Managing Medical Cost Inflation

As I've mentioned before, Hillary Clinton deserves significant credit for the slowing of health care costs. During the height of the national health care reform debate, the threat of wholesale national reform intimidated many health care providers into being much more thoughtful and careful in their utilization of services. Since that time, we've seen an upturn in medical loss ratios (the proportion of the insurance premium going to direct caregiving), which reflects that medical costs are on the rise again. A significant proportion of this increase has to do with the utilization and pricing of drugs, but across a wide spectrum of indicators—whether it be intensity of utilization, number of visits, bed days per thousand, or total cost—overall utilization in the health system increased in 1997 and 1998. Part of this change undoubtedly reflects the slow processes of demographics, but demography alone cannot explain these upturns in utilization. Aging per se has a very small impact on utilization; this can be easily documented. If you take age-specific utilization rates (for example the number of office visits per capita for sixty- to seventy-year-olds today) and multiply them by future census age cohorts (for example the number of sixty- to seventy-year-olds year olds in 2020), you can calculate the pure aging effect. It is about 1 to 2 percent annually; the aging effect does not become a major effect (3 percent or more) until between 2017 to 2020.

We can see that aging per se is not the real culprit behind escalation of health costs. Rather, it is what health services researchers call upward-bending age-specific utilization rates, which in simple terms means we're doing more for the average seventy-five-year-old with disease X than we did ten years ago.

In a classic article titled "The Illusions of Necessity," Bob Evans, the Canadian health economist, pointed out that aging and technology were not in and of themselves going to cause escalation in costs. As we have discussed, aging has a small effect, and technology has an effect only if it is continuously applied. The escalation is brought about by the increase in utilization of such procedures as hip replacement and carotid endarterectomies for successively older age cohorts.

Other areas that explain the upturn in medical loss ratios include increases in costs and intensity of servicing outside the hospital, including rehabilitation services, home health care services, infusion therapy, and respiratory therapy. A further area in which escalation has occurred is in rural medicine. According to George Halvorson, CEO of Health Partners, an HMO based in Minneapolis, his HMO paid three to four times more for procedures in rural areas compared to the cost of the same procedures in Minneapolis. Rural hospitals have monopolies in many instances, and they price their procedures according to whatever the market will bear.

As medical loss ratios have risen, HMOs have tried to insulate themselves by carving out deals with providers on a fixed capitation basis rather than on a percentage-of-premium basis. Capitation is good for an HMO when premiums are rising; percent of premium is good when premiums are falling. And as we see rates escalate in 1999 and beyond, it will be interesting to see how much of the rate increase trickles down in the form of increased medical loss ratios. It is not likely to be as much as providers might think, simply because the HMOs are having to dig themselves out of the hole in which they ended up as the underwriting cycle turned nasty and as losses became more prevalent.

Seeking Economies of Scale: Virtual Single Payer

Health care is a local good, and far and away the most successful HMO strategy to date has been to become what I have called a virtual single payer. This means becoming the largest player in a particular metropolitan area or state, whereby the HMO reaps not only administrative efficiencies but also increasing market power over doctors and hospitals. Administrative efficiencies are more real for health plans than for doctors, even though many HMOs that have merged have not been hugely successful in yielding administrative efficiencies. Where real efficiencies have been achieved, however, is in the clout gained over local providers.

The virtual single payer strategy delivers both on cost containment and quality (at least as measured by choice). As stated earlier, a key dimension of the public's view of quality of health care is choice of provider. A virtual single payer HMO can simultaneously offer quality, or the illusion of quality, through a broad network of providers; and because of its sheer scale and purchasing power, it can simultaneously offer low cost.

To fully exploit the virtual single payer strategy, a company must grow market share continuously, which makes this strategy consistent with one of consolidation. This has meant that the virtual single payer tends to enter all the market segments that can add lives to its firepower. Thus many of the virtual single payers participate in Medicare, Medicaid, large-group insurance, small-group insurance, Champus, HIPCs and other state employee pools if they exist, as well as some of the new aggregators, such as employee leasing organizations.

This virtual single payer strategy is really a private sector form of Canadian provincial government or of a German sickness fund, both of which in their own way coordinate purchasing power to gain control over providers' costs. It requires vigorous and aggressive negotiation by the health plan with specialists in particular.

Dr. Malik Hassan, the legendary former chairman and CEO of QualMed and then HealthNet and the Foundation Health Systems, was notorious for arriving in a white limousine to negotiate with providers in an all-or-nothing battle. The white limousine method of negotiation takes on subtler forms with other players, such as Highmark, but essentially the model is the same. It is the concentration of firepower in a few select hands and the turning of physicians into hamsters on a treadmill (as we have put it elsewhere in this book) such that their reimbursement is gradually eroded.

Virtual single payer has become the default strategy for the managed care industry, whether it be commercial insurers, such as Aetna U.S. Healthcare and Cigna; national managed care plans, such as United; or regional players that become national players, such as WellPoint and Foundation. This strategy represents the American ideal: for-profit government.

Virtual single payers frighten providers; clearly it is in providers' interest to increase the number of insurance companies so as to decrease the virtual single payer's market share and thus its purchasing clout. Therefore certain smaller insurance players have been given a break in the market to keep them in the game. For example, Blue Shield of California did not have as large a market share as some of its for-profit competitors (WellPoint, Foundation Health, and PacifiCare being the key examples). WellPoint bought second-tier players, such as Mass Mutual and John Hancock; Foundation and Health Net merged. In this oligopolistic managed care market, Blue Shield of California was accorded a competitive price from the large provider organizations (not commensurate with its market share); according to senior executives in the industry, this was done expressly because Blue Shield was a small player. In other words, players were recognizing that when it came to relieving cost containment pressure, the more payers the better. Better to give a good deal to a less dominant player than to have the market consolidate further.

Daring to Be Different

The final strategy is that of innovation and differentiation. With this strategy, a company attempts to differentiate on the basis of new products, quality, or a whole new conception of the market. Unfortunately, differentiators have not fared well in the health care market. With the commoditization of the HMO business, there has been little or no new product differentiation in HMOs in the late 1990s.

Kaiser and the group and staff model HMOs represent the mother of all differentiation strategies. Although growth of these models essentially stopped in 1990, they still have the infrastructure to demonstrate superior outcomes for a defined population. Kaiser, in California, consistently beats the HMO competition in terms of quality metrics. But the public and the employers don't just value outcomes; many consumers still value health insurance as a ticket to enter the fee-for-service medical care system. For these consumers, managed care is an impediment to access. Lite managed care plans are commodities with similar networks. The only possible differentiation for consumers and employers might be on the basis of customer service.

Superior service quality has not really been rewarded. There is no health plan equivalent of the level of customer service that United Airlines offers its passengers who fly over one hundred thousand miles per year. Do you really want to reward your frequent fliers if you're an HMO? It's quite the reverse. Declaring it treats HIV/AIDS patients better than its competitor is not in the HMO's interest; it is rewarded when it attracts the healthy, not the sick.

Similarly, those who have tried to differentiate on the basis of consumer focus and customer service, such as Oxford Health

Plans, have run into trouble by getting ahead of the market or by failing to execute, which has been the fatal flaw for many of the product innovators who have pursued this strategy. Their idea was good, but they simply couldn't execute to differentiate themselves.

Perhaps the best example of an organization that has successfully differentiated itself is Blue Shield of California. Under the leadership of CEO Wayne Moon, Blue Shield has transformed itself from being a rather sleepy kissing cousin of the more aggressive Blue Cross of California. The old Blue Shield clung valiantly to the not-for-profit banner. The new Blue Shield still does. But it has also bet the farm on a consumer orientation, providing superior trade-up service to those more affluent and discerning segments of the California population who want high-end managed care. Obviously Blue Shield cannot let its rates get too far out of line, but it can charge a little more for what is positioned as a consumer-friendly product. And because of their long-standing origins as a physician-sponsored organization, they enjoy superior relationships with doctors compared to some of the other health plans. From a marketing standpoint, Blue Shield, with its Access Plus HMO model and www.mylifepath.com Web site, has done an excellent job of positioning itself as consumer-friendly. But most important, Blue Shield has enjoyed the luxury of being a nonprofit organization in a market where all its major competitors (except for Kaiser) are publicly traded for-profit companies. It has therefore been able to invest in information infrastructure to support this vision rather than deliver profits to shareholders.

Blue Shield is not without its own challenges in terms of customer service and operational efficiency. Point-of-service plans are notoriously difficult to administer. More choice for patients builds in more complexity into administrative systems. In a price-competitive market you still have to rightsize and downsize your administrative functions as much as anyone. Blue Shield has done this in the 1990s, but it is difficult to simultaneously provide superior customer service and engage in rightsizing and downsizing, no matter how good your consultants or your administration and management skills. So although its vision and strategy remain centrally differentiated from some of its competitors, Blue Shield, like all HMOs, has to focus its energies in the future on execution. Blue

Shield is nevertheless a good example of an organization that has tried to differentiate itself in what is increasingly a commoditized business, and certainly the successful growth of its HMO product can be attributed to good marketing differentiation in the minds of consumers, brokers, and employees.

PacifiCare has tried to differentiate itself over the years, first in its focus on the Medicare market, and second as a provider-friendly partner interested in retaining enrollees for the long haul. Pacifi-Care placed heavy emphasis on retention in its strategy over the last few years by rewarding and enforcing customer satisfaction and quality. It did this through its kinder, gentler relationships with its provider partners and through incentives for both its executives and its physician partners, embodied in compensation packages that were tied to standardized customer satisfaction measures. Paci-fiCare remains a leader in the Medicare HMO market and will continue to be the pioneer in managed care for Medicare.

Differentiating on Quality

The attempts by PacifiCare and others to reward quality and service are important harbingers of possible innovation in reimbursement in the future. Fee for service at its core is an incentive to do more, whereas capitation is an incentive to do less. New forms of performance-related reimbursement—such as payment based on a combination of productivity, clinical outcomes, and customer satisfaction measures—will likely emerge in the future. The ten-year forecast of health care produced by the Institute for the Future for the Robert Wood Johnson Foundation points to the rise of performance reimbursement as a likely important innovation in future health plans, accounting for anywhere from 20 to 25 percent of all reimbursement by 2010. The precise nature of this type of reimbursement remains cloudy. It will certainly involve increased use of quality metrics and outcome measurement as a basis for reimbursement of physicians, hospital systems, and HMO executives themselves. It will also involve, as it has in the early manifestations of this model of reimbursement, feedback from consumers about their satisfaction with the plan. The precise format could even go so far as to constitute a new form of fee for service, a graded fee schedule whereby individual physicians could be moved to a higher fee depending on their quality scores and customer satisfaction measures. For example, the HMO would pay a physician a base fee of $25 for an office visit, but that fee could rise to $40 over time if quality was demonstrated (based on customer satisfaction parameters and outcomes measurements). This idea may be inherently appealing to doctors who really like taking tests, are incredibly competitive, are used to being in the top of their class, and fundamentally believe in fee for service as a mechanism for reimbursement. In this scenario, one could imagine that the physician fee schedule, instead of negatively ratcheting down over time as it does in Germany and Canada, could possibly ratchet upward in the U.S. context, depending on quality, productivity, and performance.

But before physicians go ripping up their capitation worksheets or their old fee schedules, they should be reminded that the likelihood of this scenario happening in the short run is almost zero, simply because HMOs have been more comfortable with wielding the blunt instrument of virtual single payer—near monopoly power over a captive provider community. Similarly, physicians have been reluctant to fully embrace competitive scoring on the basis of quality and cost. It may be the right and logical thing to do, and consumers will eventually demand it, but there is a lot of resistance. To date, attempts to measure such parameters at the fine-grain physician level have been thwarted by indifference on the part of both health plans and providers.

For example, the Medical Quality Commission (MQC), run by Dr. Alan Zwerner, was a group spun off from the Unified Medical Group Association of Southern California. The MQC was intended to foster quality metrics and management within the medical group community, but it had to abandon the field of medical group quality assurance for lack of support both from providers and from the health plan sponsors who underwrote the organization. The organization couldn't sustain itself because it was too difficult to find anyone willing to foot the bill for the measurement activity. Although there is a good deal of rhetoric around increased interest in quality metrics and management, no one seems to want to pay for it.

The National Committee on Quality Assurance (NCQA) has long struggled with this problem. The NCQA leadership fully understands that quality measurement needs to move from an accreditation model to a performance measurement model based on outcomes—but try getting paid for doing performance measurement based on outcomes. The only way the NCQA can continue to be in the phone book is if it provides a unique stamp of approval, using accreditation as a vehicle for enabling it to extract some kind of levy from its HMO constituents. It is very difficult for the NCQA to abandon accreditation without finding some mechanism to sustain itself financially through performance measurement activity. The declared strategy that NCQA president Margaret O'Kane and her colleagues are pursuing makes perfect sense: migrate to performance measurement by incorporating more sophisticated measures into accreditation standards. As more clinical performance variables are added, the NCQA will move farther from measuring the structural characteristics or institutional capacities of the organization under review (which is the basis for their current accreditation programs) and closer to a system in which there is continuous monitoring (using outcomes data) of the organization's clinical and health impact.

This shift is easier said than done, and the NCQA and other organizations, such as the Foundation for Accountability (FACCT) and JCAHO, are increasingly working together in this area where they were once fierce rivals. Their combined success is vitally important. If health care and managed care are going to develop and thrive, the field needs to have referees. As managed care consolidates, it is even more important to have strong referees who are speaking with one voice.

Refereeing Quality

The growth of the managed care industry has been paralleled by the creation of an entire industry—the health care quality industry—to measure and monitor managed care. In addition to the not-for-profit pioneers in the field, namely, NCQA, FACCT, and JCAHO, there are employer coalitions, such as the Pacific Business Group on Health, not to mention armies of health benefit consultants. Part of the problem with the quality industry is that it has become just that. Until recently, more energy was put into competing with other quality measurement folks than into strengthening the movement as a whole. The quality pioneers (such as NCQA) should be excepted from this criticism because they are not making money out of being in the quality industry. But even the pioneers create added administrative burden for the managed care industry in general and physician groups in particular. For example, the typical medical group with multiple HMO contracts is required in the NCQA accreditation process to provide clinical information, chart review, and documentation for each HMO. A typical medical group may have five to ten such contracts, which causes a significant duplication of effort.

Government Regulation Versus Voluntary Industry Self-Assessment

In the debate over who should oversee quality in managed care is a tension between regulation versus voluntary industry self-assessment; that tension is profound, and it will continue to grow over the next decade. The level of government regulation seen in managed care during the early years of the new century will be highly influenced by the distribution of power between the political parties. Stronger government regulation is clearly likely to emerge if the Democrats regain the White House in 2000 and there is significant Democratic representation in Congress; in this situation, it's likely that managed care will be a much more regulated industry. If, however, a Republican Congress holds sway, then managed care is more likely to be governed in a more self-regulatory way, which might be more appropriate for an industry that still needs to be in continuous transition.

It would be a big mistake to use regulation to lock in the current best practices of HMOs as the end-state for managed care. We need to keep innovating. There is no question that politicians seem enamored with the notion of increased regulation of managed care. It doesn't seem to cost them much, and that's politically attractive. But in reality, if managed care were to be more tightly regulated, who would do it, how would it be done, and how would the important pioneering work of NCQA, FACCT, JCAHO, and others be incorporated into some kind of regulatory mechanism? A patient bill of rights would require enforcement, enforcement would require monitoring, monitoring would require standards, and standards would require the kinds of activities the NCQA and others have been engaged in. Who exactly is going to do this? One option is to give the NCQA and the other organizations deemed status so that the HCFA does not reinvent the wheel and so that the government doesn't have to re-create the kinds of infrastructure and tools for quality assessment that have already been developed. This idea may be an appropriate middle path; many state governments already use the NCQA process for HMO accreditation.

The more extreme alternative is to set up an independent organization (similar to the Securities and Exchange Commission, which oversees the securities and investment industry) for oversight of the managed care industry, which may then use contractor organizations like the NCQA. At the greatest extreme is a creation of HCFA II, a government organization intended to monitor quality and clinical outcomes. For any of these interventions to be fair, they would need to monitor and evaluate managed care and fee-for-service indemnity medicine on an equal footing.

As has been discussed elsewhere in this book, one of the central challenges the managed care industry has to face in the future is measuring quality and customer responsiveness; finding a common ground in dealing with this challenge will be extremely difficult. (The authoritative text on the quest for accountability in managed care is *Demanding Medical Excellence*, by Michael Millensen.)

The Future of Quality

Looking ahead, what do we mean by quality? Are we really interested in improving health status, or do we actually only want to make sure that medical care is monitored appropriately? The danger in all of these quality measurement systems is that we may not like the results of our measurements. If certain HMOs have demonstrably superior outcomes compared to others, what will we do with that information. Will we close down the poor performers? What if the fee-for-service insurance plans have the worst quality? Will we close them down? What if it is the Medicare system that has the worst quality? In the past, for example, the technology assessment literature proved that coronary care units were really a waste of time, yet they were rapidly diffused throughout U.S. health care because cardiologists and others were convinced they were superior. Our problem in the United States is often that we choose to ignore evidence that medical care is ineffectual and go ahead and diffuse the technology and encourage its use regardless of the scientific evidence (another example being the overuse of fetal monitoring). A parallel may exist with quality measurement. We may end up expending enormous amounts of money in developing a regulatory apparatus to monitor and measure managed care plans and end up ignoring the results.

One of the great tragedies may be that we produce these quality metrics and we don't act on them. The health care quality industry may become analogous to J.D. Powers, which is often held up as the light of all consumerist information, or to *Consumer Reports,* produced by the Consumers Union. When it comes to cars or appliances or lawnmowers, the American public systematically ignores *Consumer Reports.* We don't just go out and buy what they tell us to. Although these publications have considerable sway among their constituencies, not all Americans behave as if they've read *Consumer Reports.* Clearly, this pattern would repeat itself in health care. A better-informed public, armed with this consumer information, will still reserve the right to visit a doctor who has better bedside manner and a lousy clinical outcome. Our own preferences and experience will shape how we use this information. Similarly, will employers systemically analyze this information and use it to contract with particular health plans? Will the employees use the information in their decisions? To date, quality metrics have had more value for health benefit consultants and sophisticated employers than they have for employees and consumers.

Technical Challenges in Measuring Quality

There are also very difficult technical issues in the area of quality measurement. For example, what endpoints are we going to use to judge quality? Will they be solely clinical? Will they be related to quality of life? Will they be mortality, morbidity? Will there be broadly defined health status indicators? The endpoint you use shapes the way in which you evaluate the success of a system. I have argued that the endpoint used to judge a clinical outcome is a function of the affluence of the individual or society that is doing the judging. For example, in Bangladesh the endpoint of interest is mortality. In the United Kingdom it's morbidity. In Canada, mobility is perhaps the endpoint. In France it's quality of life because the French are obsessed with their livers and their sexual functions. And in the United States, Americans just want to *feel good*, which explains why I call this relationship between affluence and endpoint the *James Brown Effect*. But there is some truth to my "feel good" claim, because the recent blockbuster drugs that have come on the market have tended to focus on what I call the four I's: immobility, ignorance, impotence, and incontinence. Along with hosts of new anti-inflammatories are impotence medications, such as Viagra; incontinence drugs that have moved into the top ten in the last two years; and drugs for improving mental functions of various types, whether they treat schizophrenia, depression, or migraine. These are all reputedly going to be incredible commercial successes because they speak to the angst of the baby boomers and deal with some of the ailments around the four I's that the boomers are experiencing or anticipating.

A final set of quality issue relates to difficulties with the metrics and measurement of quality:

- *No good data.* Part of the problem in the quality industry is that there really aren't good data. Claims data are flawed. Encounter data are not kept routinely by HMOs to emulate claims data. Everyone wants to do outcomes analysis, but there is no continuous medical record available with all the information necessary to measure the outcomes involved.

- *Lack of electronic infrastructure.* The data sets are not well organized. There's no linkage among data sets. Privacy laws and competitive concerns prevent these data from being available to HMOs or researchers. The electronic infrastructure for standardized collection and reporting of clinical data is at very early stages of development. The quality industry has an infrastructure problem that a recent NCQA report refers to as being not insurmountable but certainly a challenge.

The overall focus on quality should be applauded. The principal value of the quality measurement industry is its attempt to improve the quality of all providers by using systematic measurement, evaluation, and feedback. No matter what, continuous quality improvement will make a contribution to raising standards. What remains to be seen is whether quality measurement will be used to differentiate individual providers or their health plans in the health care marketplace in a way that is meaningful to plan members and patients.

Chapter Ten

Health Care Providers

The Empire Strikes Back or Strikes Out?

Is health care a business or a profession? Is a hospital a community resource or a stock market investment? Can we have a health care delivery system that is high tech, high touch, and affordable? These questions reflect the schizophrenia in our values about health care delivery. We want customer responsiveness like any other business, but we want caring, compassion, and community unlike any other business. We need a new vision for health care delivery, one that moves beyond grinding down the real prices of physicians and hospitals. We need to innovate, not simply reengineer and downsize.

But there is significant inertia in the field of health care delivery. From a provider's point of view, health care is still largely about patients being treated by doctors in hospitals either as inpatients or outpatients. Spending on physicians and hospitals still accounts for two-thirds of all health spending, and much of the administrative portion of health care supports these activities. Hospitals, doctors, nurses, and the other health care professionals remain the central actors in health care. How are providers coping with the changes we have described? Are they fighting back or failing? This chapter focuses on how providers are reacting to a changing health care environment. We will explore how providers of all types are coping with this new environment. Industry transformation has been about methods of payment and control; we have done precious little to change the way health care is delivered.

Docs Behaving Badly

The only thing that is truly global about health care is that doctors are cranky everywhere. Physicians are fearful of the future. Doctors have had it with demanding patients, with formularies, with drug detailers, with group purchasing organizations, with IPA bosses, with utilization reviewers' second-guessing them, with third-party administrators, with PPM companies that promised the earth and folded, with malpractice suits, with trial lawyers, with hospital CEOs who suckered them into PHOs in the name of capitation and then left them holding the bag, with MBAs, with suits in general, and with the goddamn HMOs. Doctors have reasons to be upset.

But so far, we have not heard doctors tell us what they want the future to be. Doctors need to consider their future, because if they do not help develop some new visions for the future, if they do not show some leadership, then they can look forward to a default future that, as baseball great Goose Gossage once said, "looks a lot like the present only longer." As we have seen, if medical care doesn't change, physicians can look forward to a future of being hamsters in a treadmill. For as managed care plans increasingly behave as virtual single payers, U.S. physicians will increasingly be working under circumstances akin to those of physicians in Germany and Canada. Doctors need to envision a better future than being hamsters, a future that does not involve a return to 1975 or some other imagined past.

The 1 Percent Problem: Exploring the Possibilities of Medical Care in the New Millennium

Doctors do great stuff. They save lives and stamp out disease. They help make us well, and they assist us through the difficult life events of birth, illness, and death. As we enter the new millennium, physicians are armed with dazzling new technologies that hold the promise of radical change in prevention, diagnosis, and treatment: scanners, gene therapy, xenotransplantation, new pharmaceuticals— a whole host of new tools and technologies that will make medical care even more powerful will come on-line in the decades ahead.

The practice of medicine has changed. More doctors are in large groups (even though most doctors aren't). More doctors are employed. Almost all physicians have been affected by managed care, most of them negatively. Autonomy is down, incomes are under pressure, and doctors everywhere are cranky.

Yet despite these changes, medicine is practiced in a very tiny space. The office visit, the consultation, the history, the physical, the process of diagnosis, the referral, and the operation are all hundred-year-old ideas that have changed little. Despite the emergence of capitation and salaried models of care in HMOs, these models of payment have stalled at including less than 20 percent of all physicians. Similarly, 90 percent of doctors don't work in large group practices. Medical practice has impressive new tools but ancient models of organization and delivery of service.

There are five key dimensions for change in medical practice, and each seems set to expand as we enter the new millennium:

1. *New medical technologies* that will transform the physician's armamentarium.
2. *New information technologies,* particularly the Internet and e-commerce, that could profoundly alter the possible interactions between physicians and their patients.
3. *Consumerization of health care,* stimulated both by sophisticated new consumers demanding more and by the reluctantly empowered customers who are forced to be more consumerist by the massive shift to defined contribution taking place in health care.
4. *Reimbursement methods.* Fee for service, capitation, and salary are the only ideas around. Every other industry is developing whole new business models to serve new consumers with the new technology. The health care industry needs to invent and test new business models for medical practice.
5. *Organizational forms.* Solo, small groups, large groups, PPMs, and IPAs—the organizational forms are quite limited. Let's broaden our view of how professionals can be organized. We can learn lessons from financial services, consulting, other knowledge professions, creative professions, even the entertainment industry.

The number of possibilities for the organization and delivery of medical care will expand in each of these five dimensions. Suppose that we could double or perhaps triple the number of options available in each dimension. Cumulatively that would be at least a hundredfold increase in the possibilities for the organization of medical care. Right now we are flailing around inside 1 percent of the possible space. What follows is a start on how to get at the other 99 percent.

New Medical Technology

The new biology is at the core of the transformation under way in clinical medicine. The exposition of the human genome and the diagnostic and therapeutic tools that follow will create new opportunities for practice. Similarly, nanotechnology (microscopic machines that could conceivably clean out arteries or clip aneurisms), robotics, and the rise of alternative therapy each will have a profound impact on the tools and content of medicine. What will this mean for physicians and how they organize?

The most important effect of these new technologies will be to stimulate a reexamination of the roles that physicians play. There are likely to be six core functions that physicians will perform in the new medicine:

1. *Clinical data collector.* Physicians have certain unique data-collection skills that bring a huge amount of knowledge to bear on the sounds, sights, and images being presented to them. For example, in auscultation (using the stethoscope) a doctor gets a lot of information that a less well trained practitioner might not recognize. Similarly, physicians are likely to continue to play a role in the collection and interpretation of information derived from how patients look and feel. Increasingly, though, these clinical data-collection functions will be replaced by diagnostic probes and sensors and, in the area of imaging, by pattern-recognition computer intelligence applied to MRI and PET scanners. The role of clinical data collector may be reduced, but it won't disappear.

2. *Shaman.* Modern physicians often underestimate the power of their ancient role as healer. The shaman factor will become more important in a world of machines and digital intelligence. Birth, illness, and death are spiritual events. Physicians play an important ceremonial role in these events, whether they recognize

it or not. Part of the reason for the rapid growth in alternative and complementary medicine in recent years is that people are thirsting for a spiritual connection to their healers.

3. *Health adviser and wellness coach.* Compliance is a huge issue in medical care. People know they shouldn't do most of the unhealthy things that taste and feel good, but they do them anyway. Patients don't take medications even when they work. We don't listen. Actually, doctors have huge persuasive power; they just don't often use it on the right subject. For example, physicians are notorious for not exploring and addressing substance abuse (alcohol, tobacco, and narcotics). Physicians could be powerful health and wellness coaches if they harnessed their knowledge to the new information technology. For example, imagine having your own digital date with your doctor every day. Every day, you get an e-mail from your doctor with some key questions, reminders, and data-collection points. The e-mails are computer generated and the responses analyzed automatically, but if you falter you get periodic voice mails, summons to your physician's office, even house calls. Imagine how healthy we would be. The worried well could be soothed electronically. Of course, much of this could be achieved *without* doctors, which is no doubt one reason why doctors are worried about changing.

4. *Knowledge navigator.* Harris surveys showed that sixty million Americans went on-line in 1998 for health care information and that 91 percent of those found what they were looking for. Problem solved, right? Not quite. Despite the explosion of health information on-line, despite the FAQs and all the search engines, access to information without the knowledge to process it can make people more uncertain and confused. Increasingly, we will have patients and families with huge amounts of information but little knowledge. They will need help and coaching in managing, interpreting, and customizing information about health and disease. Physicians potentially could be the perfect knowledge navigators, helping patients through difficult choices by helping them develop customized decision trees on treatment, by coaching on sources, and by advising on when knowing more may be bad for your health and well-being. There will be technology-based solutions that will purport to synthesize, but again, doctors are uniquely qualified to harness the new tools to serve patients.

5. *Proceduralists.* Despite nanotechnology, robotics, noninvasive surgery, and advances in pharmacology, there will still be a lot

of scoping, groping, probing, and even cutting done in the new millennium. Doctors will have a big part to play in the residual of twentieth-century medical care that spills over into the twenty-first. And remember, physicians have never run out of things to do. When antibiotics largely eliminated tuberculosis and the sanitaria that served those patients, physicians didn't just disappear from the field. The new proceduralists will be nanosurgeons (no *Mork and Mindy* jokes please), digital radiologists, invasive geneticists, and xenotransplant surgeons.

6. *Diagnostician.* Every nonmedical person imagines a future in which diagnosis is performed by machines. Samples are drawn, tests are run, results are analyzed, diagnosis is calculated—all by a thing that looks like a Palm Pilot or, even better, by subcutaneous sensors connected wirelessly to America Online. This has been the future for more than thirty years—on *Star Trek* alone. When Technicon developed the twenty-channel blood chemistry analyzer in the 1960s, many believed that a simple battery of tests was all you needed to diagnose most problems. Some went as far as to advocate multiphasic screening of whole populations using the new technology. Well, there was a snag: the tests were not perfectly sensitive or specific, which resulted in enormously high numbers of false positive and false negative results. We must be careful we don't fall into a similar but more sophisticated technological trap. Physicians will still play a critical role in synthesizing a wide variety of data inputs within a knowledge and decision-making framework that is tough to emulate on even our most powerful computers. But doctors would be wrong to assume that they will never be replaced as diagnosticians. Rather, some physicians who learn to use the new tools will make quantum improvements in the quality and productivity of diagnosing disease—perhaps edging out their less-savvy colleagues.

The Internet and E-Commerce

The century of digital technology is upon us, and its greatest manifestation is the Internet. The Internet and e-commerce are transforming every business they touch. But first, remember Morrison's Five Laws of the Internet:

LAW 1: The Internet Is the Mother of All Commoditizers

E-commerce eats margin and turns everything into a commodity big time. From Priceline.com to Amazon.com, e-commerce has gutted the margin on almost every business segment it has touched. When medicine gets touched by the Internet, margin will be taken out. The first candidates for extinction in health care will be brokers and agents in the small-group insurance market, whose 10 percent take is sheer wasted motion. Channelpoint, an Internet start-up that is focused on automating the insurance brokerage function, and others will be quick to vaporize that margin. Erosion of medical care margins will follow, albeit at a slower pace.

LAW 2: The Margin That Is Eliminated Is Not Captured by the Innovator but by the Consumer

Amazon doesn't get the margin that has been taken out of the old business. This is kamikaze kapitalism. The company loses money but changes the world for the better. In health care the new e-commerce innovators will make money in IPOs, to be sure, but the Healtheons of the world may change the rules of the game without ever capturing the margin for themselves.

LAW 3: The Web Is a One-to-One Medium, but the Race Is on to Build Killer Mass Brands

The Internet is about one-to-one marketing. It enables pluralism to thrive. But the business race is on to be the number one or two e-businesses in each segment. Huge valuations will be given to the winners in on-line trading, browsers, portals, sports centers, retailing, auctions, you name it. In health care the race is on to own the physician's desktop (duh—physicians don't work at desks), to own the on-line pharmacy business, to be the medical portal, and to be the content leaders in a particular disease area. Companies like Web MD will spend a fortune to establish market preeminence regardless of revenue or profitability. This point leads us to the fourth Law.

LAW 4: Internet Advertising Is Like the Alberta Tar Sands

Canadians are proud that there is the equivalent of two Middle East's–worth of oil in the Alberta tar sands. There's just one wee problem. The amount of energy it takes to extract the oil exceeds the amount of energy produced by the oil extracted. You have to put in more than you get out, indefinitely, until something fundamentally changes with the technology. And so it is with Internet advertising. Every major Internet player, with the exception of AOL and Yahoo!, spends more on advertising costs than it collects in advertising revenues. This situation may well continue in perpetuity. In health care, the innovators will spend a fortune to establish brands. There will be continued escalation in health care advertising by not only pharmaceutical companies but also hospitals and, most important, the emerging e-commerce players.

LAW 5: There Is a Huge Amount of Physical Fulfillment in E-Commerce

Most e-businesses are crude versions of the following scenario: we'll sell you a $20 book for 40 percent off and then FedEx it to you for $10. Many of the e-commerce players are logistically challenged, staffed with Seattle snowboarding stoners stumbling around in badly organized warehouses. And this is scalable? In health care, the patient or a physical specimen has to be involved in a lot of health care transactions, and this is likely to be the case for a very long time. (Trust me—it was my Ph.D. thesis.)

E-commerce is a vicious, wonderful thing. It will transform health care to the benefit of consumers and to the lucky few founders and early investors in the true innovators. Properly applied, e-commerce can yield enormous benefits in creating greater connectivity, quality, consistency, and customization of medical practice. It will enrich the experience for the consumer if not for the provider.

Consumerization

Health care is being consumerized. Not in the way some describe, with gleeful Valley Girl consumers shopping for medical care the way they shop at the mall: "Oh ma God, I found a fabulous new surgeon, 30 percent off." Certainly some sophisticated consumers are trading up with their own money, but the vast majority of consumerism is being driven by two key factors. First is the skepticism and dissatisfaction with traditional medical care and managed care

processes of care; people don't like gatekeepers and specialty referral restrictions and the fact that doctors are so harried by managed
care that they don't have time to spend with patients. (Welcome to
HamsterCare.) The second likely factor is the emergence of a new
consumer group—the reluctantly empowered. These are people
who have been forced by the shift from defined benefit to defined
contribution by employers and the Medicare program to be more
consumerist in their interaction with health plans and providers.

The Internet is an amplifier of consumerization. Armed with
new technologies and empowered, the consumer is going to want
to interact with physicians in very different ways.

New Reimbursement Models

Currently there is a spectrum of reimbursement methods from fee
for service through fee per episode and capitation, all the way to
salaries in a global budget environment. Generally speaking, the
closer you move toward global budgets, the more contained your
overall health care costs will be, even though individual physicians'
productivity (and incomes) will be much less. We need new reimbursement ideas.

In a *Health Forum Journal* article ("Leadership and White Space:
The Struggle for Strategy Innovation in Healthcare," May-June
1999), I identified the following possibilities for reimbursements
in the future:

• *Micro fee for service.* Many sophisticated consumers want a
quick answer from their doctor. Sure, nurse advice lines are great,
but sometimes patients want an answer from their physician. Why
can't we have microtransactions? For example, doctors could get
paid a micro fee for service by patients who hit on the FAQ section
of their physician's Web site. Doctors could get paid a micro fee
for service for answering e-mails and voice mails from patients.
Doctors could make electronic house calls using videoconferenc-
ing and telemetry and charge micro fees for service.

• *Group and community visits.* Many patients have chronic conditions; they need a lot of teaching and dialogue about their disease and about the consequences for daily living. Sometimes the
office visit is not the best model for imparting this information. Why
are there not more group and community teaching and serving

opportunities? For example, there could be diabetic day clinics in which internal medicine specialists, nephrologists, nurses, and dietitians engage a patient group in a dialogue about their illness and its treatments, fifteen or thirty patients at a time. Research by Ed Noffsiger and his colleagues at Kaiser Permanente has shown spectacular clinical results and improved patient satisfaction with two-hour drop-in visits during which fifteen to twenty cancer patients meet with a physician and other professionals together in a group. The patients love it, the doctors love it, and outcomes have improved substantially. According to Kaiser, the limiting factor is physical space for such meetings. The traditional examination room would get a little crowded.

Along similar lines, why can't a doctor be paid for being a sysop: a host in a chat room where he or she tends a chronically ill flock electronically? We need compensation schemes to make these types of encounters a reality.

• *Physician as personal health coach.* Many consumers want their health providers to take a holistic view of health. Physicians could be coaching and advising more than diagnosing and treating. We need reimbursement schemes and health plans that offer the opportunity for longer coaching interactions.

New Organizational Forms

The organization of medicine has changed little in a century. The idea of the large multispecialty group practice, whether on the Mayo model or the Permanente model, is at least fifty years old, and far from mainstream. The modern model—the IPA—is perfect for physicians in that it allows them to preserve their autonomy yet huddle together for warmth, and, most important, it doesn't force them to commit to one organization. It is a perfect model for organizationally challenged, passive-aggressive loners. Similarly, another effort at organizational reform—the PPM companies—were run by unfortunate businesspeople who thought medicine was an easy play to rationalize. Wrong, you lose.

Where can physicians look for new models? Here are four possibilities:

• *Consulting companies.* The Big Five accounting firms and the large consultants have tens of thousands of employees and thousands of partners. The Permanente model is closest to this format, but the consultants have learned lessons even Permanente has not yet fully developed: the importance of standards, training, and pyramids. Most big consulting companies have standardized their technology platforms and systems, their knowledge assets, and their business processes nationally and globally. No one in health care has done this with physicians on any sort of scale. In terms of training, for example, Andersen Consulting and Arthur Andersen share the St. Charles facility, a two-thousand-room former women's college outside Chicago, which trains and upgrades the skills of tens of thousands of Androids every year. The investment in training by the combined firm is gigantic—upwards of 7 percent per annum, unlike any player in medicine, even Permanente.

The biggest lesson learned by the Big Five is the power of the pyramid: senior partners make much more in compensation than they can bill as individuals; they earn based on the value created by the people who work for them. Leveraging the labor of others has never been physicians' strong point, with the exception of a few diagnostic plays, such as clinical labs. Where are the physician practices in which leading talented doctors build and lead teams of other talented physicians and other health care professionals?

- *Creative agencies.* In design, advertising, architecture and planning, and a whole host of creative professions, firms are built by melding the skills of a disparate set of creative people. They function in interdisciplinary teams where there is no superior-subordinate relationship among the skill sets.

- *Movie model.* Film crews, directors, producers, and cast come together around individual projects with a budget. Imagine that patients become projects: directors and producers assemble the best resources—free agents all—to solve clinical problems. Teams could be built using established crews or subunits as well as stars and specialists. The teams could be formed and reformed virtually as well as actually.

- *The Scottish clan model.* A variant on the movie model, this is what we might call the physician-branded PPO network. Like members of a Scottish clan, physicians develop formal kinship networks that they promote to the public on the basis of quality, performance, and value. Unlike the PPO in which the insurer selects the doctors, in this model the physicians select who they want to hang with organizationally. This is *not* the county medical society model; in that model, the ticket to entry is a stethoscope and a checkbook. In the Scottish clan model there is deep clinical respect and the willingness to ostracize and eliminate anyone who doesn't share the values and who doesn't make the grade. Permanente is the closest I've seen to this form; I am amazed that no one has tried to do it more virtually, with groups of respected colleagues branding themselves as superior. IPAs operate more on the Any Willing Schmuck model.

If You Don't Like It, Change It

Changes in the five dimensions we have examined will force physicians to rethink the way they practice medicine and to move out of the 1 percent space in which they currently conceive their work. Unfortunately, academic medical centers—the places from which we get our doctors—are among the most conservative institutions on the planet. A new cadre of Net-enabled children are heading for medical school; maybe they will change the way doctors are trained.

The ideas I have described here are a start on a bigger journey of transformation. (I'm a geographer. What do I know?) I urge doctors to think about how medicine ought to be practiced differently in the next millennium. If you don't like these futures, invent your own. Remember: 99 percent of the opportunities are unexplored.

The Next Malpractice Crisis

If managed care was not enough, if virtual single payer and hamster care were not enough, doctors may also have to deal with a new malpractice crisis. Malpractice used to be the issue that vexed doctors even more than managed care. It may do so again, because the recent lull is an anomaly. Significant progress was made in the malpractice arena in the late 1980s. Malpractice underwriters missed a significant downward inflection point in the claims rate in the mid-1980s, which caused them to overestimate the number of future claims. This fact, coupled to tort reforms in the late 1980s in California and other states, which limited the awards for pain and suffering, led to substantial underwriting surpluses for the mainstream provider-owned malpractice insurers in the late 1980s and early 1990s. These surpluses have been used to insulate providers from increases in malpractice premiums. However, three trends in combination may lead to significant escalation in malpractice insurance rates for physicians. First, claims ratios have returned to their historic normal levels. Second, there is a trend in several states (most notably Illinois) toward undoing some of the state tort reforms that placed limits on damages. Third, the AMA supports efforts by U.S. trial lawyers to bring HMOs out from under the ERISA protection against malpractice suits. Leaders in the malpractice insurance industry (which is composed principally of physician-owned mutual companies as well as a few specialized commercial carriers) anticipate that these trends will lead to a significant escalation in malpractice insurance rates over the 1999 to 2005 time period.

Malpractice is an issue that incenses physicians. A significant increase in rates, like that of the early 1980s, will coincide with increases in the hassle factor in their practice, reduced fee schedules in both Medicare and commercial insurance markets, and increased overhead of running a practice brought about by the rise of managed care. As consumers get better informed about care, and use the Internet more as a research tool, malpractice claims are likely to rise.

Malpractice is an incendiary issue for doctors, not only because the cost of insurance comes straight out of their bottom line but also because malpractice deeply affects physicians' psyche. Doctors' fear of being sued is disproportionate to actual legal or financial consequences. For example, officials of the medical malpractice insurance trade group, the Physician Insurance Association of America (PIAA), estimate that only 30 percent of malpractice suits end up in any malpractice claim against insurance. Most cases are considered frivolous. But malpractice suits irritate physicians because they put them up against their arch enemy: lawyers.

Academic Medicine and the Pursuit of Fame

The real purpose of the academic medical center is to make two people famous. Most academic medical centers are run for the benefit of a few select, premier researchers, and the goal of the entire institution is to get a Nobel Prize or two. This goal sets up a gigantic academic pyramid. To win the Nobel Prize you have to write enormous numbers of articles for the *New England Journal of Medicine* or for *Science*. To do that, you need time, talent, and money; if you don't have any time and you don't have any talent, you can make up for it with money.

In turn the money is generated through service, education, and research itself. In turn, the funds that flow to support those activities come from the following sources:

- Philanthropy, which makes up only a very small part.
- Tuition, which despite enormous increases over the last twenty years still makes up only a quarter to a third of the funding of the typical academic medical center.
- Research and government grants, which have increased recently with the doubling of National Institutes of Health (NIH) budgets.
- Faculty practice plans, through which salaried physicians give up some of their gross billings to the university in return for an opportunity to be one of the two people who get the Nobel Prize. These plans account for 40 percent of all academic medical center funding and are really the key source of funding.

This view of the academic medical enterprise may be a somewhat cynical one. However, it is a view backed up by a survey of university deans of medicine conducted for the Robert Wood Johnson Foundation by Louis Harris, which showed that research (not education and service) was the number one priority for medical schools. Moreover, the study suggested that many deans felt that this focus on research was at the expense of clinical service and teaching.

In fairness to the academic medical centers, they have been the pioneer reformers in transformation of the health care system in terms of training new cadres of leadership, as sources of new technologies, and as major actors in challenging the conventional medical establishment. However, they are the organizations in U.S. health care most disconnected from market forces and least knowledgeable about market dynamics. Many organizations focus on the arcana of medical politics. As one faculty member once told me, the reason why the fights in academia are so acrimonious is that the stakes are so low.

The typical academic medical center has a senate and other internal political processes that insulate it from rational decision making in response to the marketplace. The medical curriculum is perhaps the most competitive environment, as various organizations and faculty members vie for a share of physicians' time and training. For example, pharmacologists, health economists, nutritionists, internists, and psychiatrists jockey for more time on the medical curriculum. The poor interns and residents who go through the process become indentured servants for several years, their labor being used as part of the billing machine to support the enterprise generally. Despite the fact that these organizations have produced high-quality personnel for the U.S. health system, they have been singularly out of touch with the demands of the health care marketplace. The number of specialists continues to rise even though the demand in the marketplace is for more primary care physicians. Subspecialty positions continue to escalate—more neurosurgeons, more ophthalmologists—even though the market indicates that the demand for these professions is going to decline as managed care grows.

The managed care industry has been unwilling to cross-subsidize academic medicine the way insurers have in the past. Indeed, there is a significant degree to which managed care, though not intent on killing the academic medical center, has insisted that it would rather contract with community-based organizations that do not have the teaching overhead.

One could argue that academic medicine should prefer to have a separate set of ledgers with specific funding targeted for the educational component rather than being buffeted by an uncertain managed care marketplace. However, lobbying organizations of the mainstream academic medical centers have argued quite the reverse, preferring to hide under the umbrella of service upgrades for complexity, teaching factors, upgrading their DRG funding, and so forth. They do this because it's easier to hide their research budget under the cloak of service. By hiding under one consolidated budget, the academic medical center can cross-subsidize to create the Nobel Prize winners. If the true costs of research were isolated as a separate line item with explicit funding, academic medicine would run the risk of being managed politically from Washington.

It might be better for academic medicine to go this route of separate funding. Certainly surveys indicate that the American public is incredibly supportive of medical research and think it's the highest priority of all among the various areas of research spending. Framed as a research and innovation issue, the whole notion of the academic pyramid might be quite appealing to the general public as a federally funded separate set of institutions. Yet mainstream academic medicine seems to be reluctant to take the risk of being carved out in this fashion.

The multiple missions of the academic medical center are at odds with managed care. In particular, academic medicine is simultaneously trying to

- Create excellence in research
- Teach the new generation of providers
- Provide clinical service, particularly for complex and esoteric diseases, using advanced medical technology

All of these goals are at odds with managed care. Managed care is increasingly going to be in conflict with academic medical centers, forcing them to change their behavior one way or another. A good example of how centers have responded to the threat of managed care is the case of Stanford and UCSF: although they have not combined their medical schools, they have combined their hospitals under one organization, UCSF Stanford Health Care. This merger has been successful in creating a monopoly on quaternary services in Northern California. Its recent financial problems stem from competition in the less esoteric care sector. Similarly, Health Partners in Boston (the merger of Brigham and Women's Hospital and Massachusetts General Hospital) have created a substantial institution that has enormous market clout in the Boston environment.

Leaders of these organizations comment that at least the mergers have gotten the attention of their clinical staff so that they are a little more circumspect in their demands for resources internally, recognizing that some form of clinical rationalization has to take place in the name of institutional survival.

Hospitals: Community Resource or Pawns in the Business of Health?

Hospitals have had uneven financial performance in the late 1990s. Roughly a third of hospitals are doing well, with operating margins as high as 10 percent or more according to industry insiders; a third are hanging on, with operating margins in surplus in the mid-1990s but turning negative in the late 1990s, at least for patient care activities; and a third are doing extremely badly and are constantly struggling financially. Many hospitals remain in the black solely because of a booming stock market that allows them to make up in investment income what they lose in operations. The Balanced Budget Act provisions of 1997 hurt hospitals by cutting back future Medicare reimbursement. Part of the reason that hospital reimbursement rates were cut is that policymakers looked at the *average* net margin of hospitals—a healthy 4-plus percent—rather than at the third of hospitals in trouble and the other third put into trouble by the Balanced Budget Act cutbacks. Those hospitals that survive and prosper in the future will be those that carve out geographic monopolies or areas of specialization that allow them to differentiate themselves.

Strategic Menu for Health Care Providers

The provider sector has a strategic menu similar to the health plans in terms of growth, margin, and sustainable, defensible positions.

Acquisition Machines

In terms of growth, the first option is to become an acquisition machine, using the leverage of balance sheets and the ability to purchase (in the case of for-profit organizations) with stock or debt rather than with cash generated through retained earnings. This is obviously the strategy pursued by Columbia/HCA in the hospital sector and by Phycor, FPA, Coastal Physicians, and MedPartners in the PPM business. Acquisition machines in the provider sector have fallen out of favor, for reasons already discussed: in particular, the lack of sustainable margin on a per-hospital or per group basis, the myth of overhead consolidation, and the simple difficulties of integrating what is an incredibly fragmented delivery system. Even with larger institutions, such as hospitals, one is still hard pressed to find the economies of scale in owning two hundred hospitals in the Sun Belt.

One clear area in which economies of scale can be developed is group purchasing, but it is not necessary to own all hospitals to avail oneself of the group purchasing model. The Voluntary Hospital Association (VHA) and Premier Health Alliance, two of the largest group purchasing organizations, have approximately $11 billion in purchasing power each. At its height, Columbia/HCA had approximately $3 billion in purchasing power, yet CEO Rick Scott convinced Wall Street analysts that he had invented some amazing proprietary advantage in the fact that he was purchasing on a group basis. Bear in mind that Wall Street analysts, despite their high level of education, are one of the two groups of Americans who don't get out enough. The other group is people in Washington. As a consequence, they are easily misled by slick-talking CEOs who come to town with a plausible idea, even though in this case, Columbia/HCA's purchasing power was a fraction of its not-for-profit VHA and Premier competitors.

Horizontal Cartels

The second strategy for growth, which has been more popular with the not-for-profit community, is to form horizontal cartels. Regional consolidation on a horizontal rather than vertical basis has given the provider sector countervailing firepower against HMOs. Significant cartels—OPEC Health Care, if you like—have emerged. Intermountain Healthcare, Presbyterian Health Systems in New Mexico, Sutter Health in California, and Catholic Healthcare West throughout the western United States are good examples of this strategy. Similar organizations have been formed in such disparate markets as Florida, Iowa, Ohio, and Oregon.

Horizontal consolidation provides countervailing negotiating power to the equally rapidly consolidating managed care plans, so oligopoly is facing oligopsony in many markets. Massive horizontal consolidation of buyers (such as CalPers or the purchasing coalition the Pacific Business Group on Health) stimulates consolidation of health plans and further stimulates horizontal—not vertical—consolidation of providers in a local area.

Local Monopolies

By far the most successful strategy for sustaining margin and defending the organization is to create local monopolies. This relates to Christaller's "central place" theory. Christaller was a wacky German geographer in the nineteenth century who argued that there's only so far you'll go to buy hay (deeply profound). He discovered that there was a significant correlation among the settlement patterns of southern Germany, which indicated that the distance people were willing to travel to market for particular goods and services dictated the size and distance between the various settlements. The same is true for medical care. You'll go two blocks for primary care, twelve blocks for specialty care, and a hundred miles for a total head transplant. There is a natural geographic catchment area for hospitals and health systems.

Hospitals that successfully dominate local markets are those that are in relatively affluent suburbs. They thus avoid Medicaid recipients and the uninsured, which keeps their charitable and uncompensated care caseloads to a minimum and allows them to aggressively pursue those well-insured patients in the community.

Similarly, as we discussed earlier in this chapter, certain academic medical centers—UCSF Stanford Health Care and Health Partners in Boston—have developed virtual monopolies of quaternary care, which allow them to survive if not flourish, because very few people actually leave their metropolitan area for health care, even for treatment of the more esoteric diseases. Even prestigious medical centers in California, such as UCSF Stanford Health Care or Cedars Sinai in Beverly Hills, get over 90 percent of their patients and revenues from within thirty miles of the hospital. For these most prestigious brand-name organizations, health care is still a local good rather than an international or national good.

There are exceptions to this generalization. The Cleveland Clinic, Johns Hopkins Health System in Baltimore, and Methodist Hospital in Dallas aggressively pursued the global health care business (seeking affluent patients from around the world). The Mayo

Clinic in Rochester, Minnesota, clearly derives a significant proportion of its revenues from referrals outside the region. Despite these notable exceptions, health care is a local good. To be a success in health care delivery, you have to be a success locally.

Upscale Branding

A second strategy for maintaining margin is upscale branding; that is, the institution positions itself as having superior clinical performance in a particular line of business. Provider branding is going to increase substantially in the future, consistent with a disease-specific focus. This is more marketing push than consumer pull. Advertising budgets for hospitals are going to increase. If one visits the annual conference of the Society for Health Strategy and Market Development, a membership group of the AHA, one is struck by the number of sophisticated marketing people being brought into the health system expressly for the purpose of stimulating demand. It is no accident, therefore, that health utilization is increasing. Institutions are competing for patient loads, volumes, and margin, and they are using sophisticated advertising and marketing techniques to increase the overall utilization of health services in their community by not only capturing share from their competitors but by stimulating among consumers a perceived need for particular health services. At a recent meeting I attended, I saw several poster demonstrations proudly proclaiming the goal of increasing utilization of a particular procedure by 5 or 10 percent. If one were to view this in a Canadian or Australian context, it would be a laughable set of initiatives. In fact, quite the reverse would be the case—there would be government-sponsored programs to reduce unnecessary utilization.

In fairness to these programs, some of the utilization stimulated may indeed be necessary, as in the cases of outreach to vulnerable populations or to people failing to comply with drug therapy. Nevertheless, the overall goal of many of these marketing programs is to stimulate overall utilization. Whether you are paid on a per diem, DRG, or fee-for-service basis, more is better. It's only when you have global budgets or capitation that more is worse. Most hospitals are not capitated or on global budgets. Considering all this marketing activity, it is questionable whether any procedure-oriented, specialty service is underutilized in the United States, except among those patients with inadequate health insurance coverage or who live in very remote areas.

Expect significant increases in advertising in the future and significant increases in marketing activity as hospitals try to develop differentiated product offerings across their service lines.

Defending the Turf: Buy the Doctors, Buy the Patients, Buy the Legislators

Hospitals have tried to sustain a defensible position using a number of strategies, including the following:

Buy the Doctors

In the early 1990s it was fashionable for hospitals to purchase physician practices, particularly family practice and internal medicine group practices, as feeders to the large hospital systems. What became clear as the prices for these practices were bid up to almost a million dollars per doctor was that buying a practice did not necessarily secure patient streams and that at those kinds of prices you couldn't buy enough doctors to fill the average hospital. By 1998, virtually every physician practice purchased by a hospital was losing money. There may be other strategic synergies (which is code for "We wish we never did this, but it's too late now"), but except for a few rare situations that I will describe below, owning doctors is a bad idea.

Hospitals' desire to purchase practices was also bid up by competition from for-profit provider chains, such as Phycor and Med-Partners. As the overall orgy of purchasing cooled, what we saw was significant devaluation of these practices and a return of these practices to private hands in the wake of a series of spectacular PPM failures.

Buying the doctors was never a particularly smart strategy. Why would you want to capitalize the future income stream of a bunch of passive-aggressive people? However, in particular markets, purchasing physician groups was a justifiable defensive move to prevent incursion by a competitor. If a physician group on the edge of your service territory is struggling to survive and is being courted by a competitor ninety miles away that sees ownership of the group as a foothold on the edge of *its* service territory, then you may have a good reason to buy. This is particularly true of those institutions pursuing a local monopoly strategy. Purchasing physicians to prevent the thin edge of a wedge being driven into your service territory is not a dumb thing to do. Similarly, in a less advanced managed care market, it may be sensible to purchase the practices of certain high-flying admitters who may have been struggling because of the initial sting of managed care utilization controls. Retaining loyalty through ownership of the practice may make sense. Certain institutions, such as Waukesha Hospital in Wisconsin, responded to the request from physicians in the community to help them sustain their practices in the face of increased competitive pressure. Waukesha, for one, was happy to assist physicians in this way, to preserve the local health care infrastructure. This is a sensible way to "own the ground" locally. Generally, however, there really wasn't as much advantage in owning physicians as the mantra of the early 1990s would have had us believe.

Looking forward, it seems that simply owning physician practices is not a strategy for insuring profitability of hospitals. Many of the transactions that took place in the 1990s were motivated by a fear of losing income, either on the part of the physicians or on the part of hospitals. Terrified by the Advisory Board and other consultants into believing the "Russians were coming," hospital executives suffered from premature extrapolation. Capitation and integration were supposed to happen by a week from Monday. In a panic, hospitals scrambled to buy primary care doctors and prepare for the inevitable wave of capitated managed care.

Capitation grows like cable TV, not color TV. Cable TV took more than thirty years to reach a 60 percent penetration of U.S. households; color TV took about three years. Hospitals behaved as if capitation were like color TV.

Buy the Patients

Hospitals have also attempted the strategy of buying the patients, namely, of getting into the HMO business. Here again it must be stressed that there is a fundamental conflict between owning and running an HMO and owning and running a hospital. The classic example was that of Equitable Insurance Company and HCA, the forerunner of Columbia/HCA; they pooled their assets in a joint venture, Equicor. But the tension among their leadership was always prevalent. Equitable was trying to empty beds while HCA was trying to fill beds. The joint entity was fundamentally, strategically schizophrenic, and it never really fully developed an ability to manage care in any coordinated way. Similarly, Humana struggled to develop a clear mission as to whether it was a managed care company or a hospital company, and it had to divest of its hospitals in large measure because the schizophrenia was unbearable.

Hospitals that have pursued this strategy of owning a local HMO—Hamot and St. Vincent's in Erie, Pennsylvania; Quorum in Stockton, California; Baptist Health Systems in Miami; and many others—have struggled because of the schizophrenia. In addition, in a discounted fee-for-service managed care marketplace they inevitably faltered, in large part because most hospital-based HMOs are missing the core competencies of marketing and underwriting, particularly sales and marketing to large and small employers that the typical HMO possesses.

Certainly, if capitation had prevailed, had the pure form of managed competition prevailed, then this strategy would have made more sense. But the strategy was part of a brief moment in the sun in hospital management, when values, theory, incentives, and strategies were aligned. Hospitals were going to care about the health of a defined population because they were at risk on a capitated basis. Moreover, hospitals were going to vertically integrate to keep utilization and costs down and also be accountable for health, not just health care; and finally, once under the integrated umbrella, we could shift resources to their highest and best use across the continuum of care: from inpatient to outpatient, from step-down to home care, from inpatient surgery to the outpatient surgery center. It was a beautiful moment, and not all that bad an idea. But, in typical fashion, we rejoiced and then moved on.

Buy the Legislators

A third defensive strategy is to influence legislators to ensure that hospitals and providers are protected from the excesses of managed care. Good examples of this strategy are legislative initiatives at the state level to regulate managed care or insist that particular providers are included in any managed care plan or in any system of care.

At a recent strategic planning session of hospital executives, I explained the strategy of buying the legislators. One executive, who had been relatively poker faced through the entire session, smiled broadly when this slide came up. I asked him why he was smiling. He said, "We bought the legislators."

Long-Term Care: Warehousing or Home Alone

Nursing homes in the United States are not the dream for the future of average baby boomers or for their parents. Most individuals aspire to living at home in a healthy environment with home care provided, as and when it is needed.

The nursing home business has been relatively flat in terms of total numbers of folk admitted to nursing homes, partly because of a supply problem, on the one hand, and partly because of a lack of insurance, on the other. The de facto long-term care policy for Americans is Medicaid, with approximately one-third of all Medicaid funding being targeted to long-term care for the elderly. Recent legislative proposals suggested that the long-term care benefit of some $7 billion would be made available. This is a drop in the bucket compared to the total long-term care bill—$7 billion is probably somewhere between 10 percent and 20 percent of the total budget required to provide a universal long-term care benefit.

Part of the difficulty in long-term care financing is the issue of moral hazard. Moral hazard is a form of insurance market failure whereby the existence of the health coverage stimulates demand for a particular service. For example, a typical eighty-year-old may have a family in their fifties from whom the eighty-year-old may receive informal care, including housing, food, shelter, and assistance with the activities of daily living. If there were a universal insurance policy available, the same elderly individual might end up in a nursing home paid for by the insurance coverage.

The moral hazard issue has always plagued the long-term care market; the market for long-term care insurance has faltered for this reason as well. A few attempts have been made to create long-term care insurance as a group benefit. Unfortunately, the nature of most of the long-term care products in the marketplace has been that of a badly structured savings plan. In other words, an actuarially fair policy is not worth buying; all it would provide is a guarantee of an income return rather than any guarantee of a covered benefit down the line. Most plans are structured to provide $100 a day of service, which is simply a guarantee of a fixed amount of money coming out at the other end of the policy, not a guarantee of covering a particular benefit. Typical buyers have tended to be closer to retirement and to the need for the service. Few young twenty-five- to forty-five-year-olds have been voluntarily attracted to this class of product. Although large companies, such as General Electric, have invested in the long-term care insurance area and anticipate long-term future growth in this business, they are starting from a very small base. Even General Electric, which claims to have the largest number of insured lives in long-term care, has no more than 300,000 insured lives. Bearing in mind that over 35 million Americans are over the age of sixty-five, this is a very small percentage of coverage by the leading market maker in long-term care insurance. Nonetheless, this market is likely to grow rapidly in the next decade, particularly if the insurance industry can develop a product that pays better than consumers buying the S&P 500 index with the premium.

Home health care has been perceived as one of the major solutions to the long-term care problem. Through the late 1980s and early 1990s, all the dimensions of home health care, including respiratory therapy, IV therapy, and home health nursing, grew in both the for-profit and not-for-profit sectors. However, by the mid-1990s, there was a substantial turnaround in the profitability of those industries and the sustainability of these programs. The industry received further shocks in 1998 with the passage of the interim reimbursement policies by the HCFA. As a stopgap measure, the provisions cut home care reimbursement rates to reduce the perceived growth and unnecessary expenditure on home health care, which was then one of the fastest-growing items of the Medicare budget. In this move, as is often the case, policy wonks confused growth in revenues with growth in margin. The margin had been declining in both the IV therapy and home health nursing businesses for several years due to competitive pressures from the managed care industry and from Medicare itself.

Home health is likely to recover in the next decade, because some rational form of prospective reimbursement will be introduced. It is in the interest of both the industry and the HCFA to find some resolution of this policy and to keep high-quality actors in the business. Hospitals have received a de facto subsidy to be in the home health business because of the way in which cost-based reimbursed Medicare home health was developed. The program allows hospitals to write off a significant part of their overhead costs at a much higher and more aggressive rate than that of commercial competitors, such as Olsten or Interim Health Services, or of other independent, not-for-profit home health agencies, such as the Visiting Nurses Association.

The reimbursement imbalance will likely be resolved over time, and home health will become more of a level playing field with predictable prospective payment. As hospitals did with DRGs, home health organizations will adjust. Two types of home health care organizations will flourish in the future. First, there will be highly competitive, for-profit organizations that develop business models that are capable of delivering clinical nursing services, IV therapy, respiratory therapy, or some combination of the three. Alternatively, many hospitals may view home health as a necessary and important contribution to the continuum of care and to the concept of an integrated system serving a whole community. There are clearly synergies and benefits to patients in having seamless relationships between physicians, hospitals, and the home health care environment. Improving the continuity of care across such programs may have a significant impact on the quality of care, particularly in the care of chronic disease and for elderly patients who are frail.

The future of this business is likely to be centrally dependent on the use of alternative technologies, including information technology, to provide support and care for patients in their home. One example is Interim Health Services and its pioneering development of the Interim In-touch phone-based system whereby patients can receive the social support they need, by accessing a central telephone operator. This is not a case of "I've fallen and I can't get up"; it's "I haven't fallen but I can't get out." There is a significant need, particularly among elderly patients, for continuous daily contact and social support. Dr. David Lawrence, CEO of Kaiser Foundation Health Plan, has stressed that social support is one of the critical missing links in building healthier communities and in providing the postacute care and continued chronic care for patients of all ages. We live in an era when families are more disintegrated, geographic mobility has separated communities, and poorer individuals are less firmly supported in their own neighborhoods. The need for social support can be met through technology, such as Interim In-touch, or by Web-based services, which help individuals keep in social contact with caregivers or with peers who are experiencing similar circumstances.

New Paradigms or Bad Ideas: The Business of Health Services

The invisible hand of capitalism got nuked by the market changes of the late 1990s. Some of the high fliers, such as PPM companies, for-profit hospital chains, and disease-state management companies, experienced spectacular reductions in earnings and in their market capitalization. Conversely, HMOs were more resilient; indeed, although many HMOs faltered, few disappeared or tanked, whereas among the PPM companies, we've seen spectacular stock declines (Coastal Physicians, MedPartners, and FPA being the most notable examples).

Roll-Ups

Why have PPM companies, in particular, faltered in the late 1990s? There are three key reasons. The first is what one might term the myth of overhead consolidation. In most industries, consolidation is a good thing because as organizations consolidate, their share going to overhead reduces with scale. Quite the reverse is true in the case of physician group practices. Medical Group Management Association (MGMA) data indicate that the larger the group, the higher the proportion of the group's revenue that goes to overhead. This increase occurs because the group starts to hire more sophisticated people and to develop more specific ways in which managerial and clinical quality can be supported, whether through purchase of information systems or use of enhanced nursing and other clinical services. The product may be better, but certainly the overhead rate is not reduced by scale.

The second key reason for the failure of PPM companies, and this is perhaps one of the less well understood dimensions of these businesses, is the desire by physicians to participate in the orgy of capitalism experienced elsewhere in the economy; in particular, doctors want access to stock options. I live in Menlo Park, California, surrounded by venture capitalists and software executives. At the typical dinner party where financial issues are discussed, doctors in our community are often frustrated that they don't have access to the kind of stock options that their Silicon Valley brethren are receiving, whether in software companies or through their venture capital relationships. So they sit around and say, "Well, I'd like to do the stock option thing."

In explaining to physicians how the market works, one needs to communicate the key notion that Wall Street values companies based on some multiple of their earnings—the price to earnings ratio (P/E). A company can expect a P/E multiple approximately equal to the growth rate in earnings of the company. In other words, if you can grow the earnings per share (EPS) of a company at 20 to 30 percent per annum, then you can be guaranteed a P/E of twenty to thirty. (In the case of Internet stocks, the projected revenue increases are in the thousands of percent and nobody worries about earnings. Revenue growth is more important than earnings. Indeed, venture capitalists argue that it is almost better to take an Internet company public with losses rather than with earnings; then you can't be called to task by such mundane issues as profitability or P/E.)

At a recent typical dinner party I overheard a doctor say, "I can do that. I'll grow my EPS by 20 to 30 percent per annum. How do I do that?" he asked.

"Well, you have to see more patients or acquire more practices."

"We can do that," he responded. "What else do we have to do?"

"Well, you have to grow your bottom line at that same rate or a little bit better."

"We can do that. How do we grow the bottom line?"

"Well, you have to keep your costs down."

"What are my costs?"

"Your income."

It was a very short conversation.

The truth is that doctors do not retain earnings either personally or professionally. They go through twelve years of sleep deprivation so they can make decisions in the middle of the night. They want the earnings now. They're not prepared to wait for those earnings, and they become concerned if they have to plough more of their excess income into retaining earnings in the practice. This is why PPM companies have been unsuccessful in really demonstrating sustained retained earnings.

Promising physicians more in terms of extracting higher prices or increased patient volume from managed care has not made up for the fact that the inherent ability to retain earnings simply doesn't exist. This is true for for-profit PPM companies and physician practices generally.

The third issue is that these PPM companies were predicated on earnings escalation based on acquisitions. In the classic Ponzi scheme sense, they used stock to make further acquisitions. Consolidations (or roll-ups as the Street likes to call them) were in favor among investors in the early 1990s. Stocks were used to purchase assets and earnings, even though there was no earnings growth on a "same-store sales" basis. (In other words, individual practices saw little growth in revenues and profitability per practice.)

In some sense the Internet plays of the late 1990s are identical to the roll-ups among PPM companies in the early 1990s. There are no earnings in many of the Internet companies, yet unlike the PPM companies their stock values are so enormous that they can actually buy real companies with real earnings. For example, @home, the fledgling cable-based Internet access provider, bought Excite for more than $6 billion, almost exactly the same amount that Ford paid for Volvo Cars. Similarly, AOL could easily buy one, if not all three, traditional broadcast networks and may do it before too long. Similarly, Yahoo!, E-Bay, and Amazon.com have sufficient market capitalization to use equity to purchase companies with real technologies and real assets. Yahoo! too could buy a major TV network. E-Bay could buy every auction house on the planet, including Christie's and Sotheby's. Amazon.com could buy every bookstore chain (although their stock would drop as a result, because selling books is a lousy low-growth business whether it's over the Net or not). In the telecom market, WorldCom parlayed an aggressive roll-up style into taking over MCI, one of the great communication properties.

In the health care arena, Columbia/HCA leveraged its balance sheet to purchase assets even though the sustained profitability on a same-hospital basis was not necessarily going to be there. PPM companies represented the extreme of nonsustainability in earnings on a "same-practice" basis, but they continued expansion in the top line. Eventually, these bubbles burst.

Disease-State Management

Disease-state management (DSM) was another high-flying idea that never really fully materialized. The idea behind DSM is that practitioners, pharmaceutical companies, health plans, and hospitals focus on optimizing the care of patients with a particular disease. The argument was that companies like American Oncology Resources would emerge focused on very specific diseases and patients and have superior clinical outcomes and cost-effectiveness because of a dedicated provider network and the use of clinical guidelines. However, in the minds of the pharmaceutical companies, DSM was really disease-state marketing. DSM was a sophisticated effort by pharmaceutical companies to get on the formulary of the managed care organizations, and once they had achieved that they had little or no interest in reducing the total cost of health care for a particular population. There were some obvious exceptions to this: Schering Plough, Smith-Kline Beacham, and others had very well documented and thought through programs for reducing the total cost and burden of disease for asthma and for diabetes. But, generally speaking, the pharmaceutical industry was more interested in using DSM as a marketing tool than as a health management tool.

On the provider side, DSM was bandied around as the next major breakthrough. There were some significant positive endeavors in the area of demand management. For example, Health Access installed nurse advice lines and call-center technology to help HMOs manage the front end of encounters with the medical profession. Such initial models were extremely helpful in affecting the interface between consumer and physician, although there are natural limits to what can be achieved through the advice-line format.

Of most interest, however, are the disease and demand management organizations centered on improving the cost-effectiveness of care for chronically ill patients. There could be tremendous potential for those organizations that have some real contribution to make in the field of managing specific, chronic conditions, such as cardiovascular disease, cancer, arthritis, and diabetes. These organizations will combine cutting-edge therapeutics with practice guidelines and integrated care plans that optimize the care of particular patients, even those with comorbidities.

The issue of comorbidity reveals one of the key fallacies in the DSM mantra. Sick people with chronic illness often have more than one disease: obese-hypertensive-diabetic is a popular combination. They don't come bar-coded—such as stand-alone diabetic—so they are difficult to typecast for standardized disease management practices and protocols. That is not to say that there isn't some feasible advantage in focusing specialty care on particular disease entities. But that care is more likely to be woven together into an integrated system by either the health plan or the provider rather than simply operating as a free-floating form of specialty organization. Magellan is an HMO that bills itself as the leading health plan in the specialty network business, focused on mental and behavioral health. Similar organizations are emerging in oncology, ophthalmology, and cardiology.

In her book *Market Driven Health Care,* Regina Herzlinger introduces the concept of the focused factory, which could possibly be a useful prescription for improving DSM. Herzlinger argues that focused factories—provider groups focused on very specific diseases or conditions—can combine superior outcomes and cost-effectiveness, as has been achieved in other service industries from hamburger chains to airlines.

There is considerable scope for improvement in the management of chronic care. Disease-specific care units will become more common, although as a general rule of thumb the more specialized a hospital gets in terms of its different units, the more likely it is to have low occupancy for each of those units, which leads to redundancy and inefficiency. As we saw in Chapter Seven, DSM and focused factories aimed at chronic care may have particular relevance for the Medicare population, because the elderly have such a high incidence of chronic conditions.

Drug Price Wars: Pharmaceuticals on a Collision Course with Managed Care and Health Care Providers

As health plans and providers struggle to be profitable, they both confront the ever increasing costs of new technology, particularly pharmaceuticals. Indeed, escalation in pharmaceutical prices and utilization is a principal reason why HMOs lost money in the late 1990s. The discontent among HMO CEOs is palpable. Some have argued that drug costs will exceed inpatient hospital costs in their commercial HMO products sometime early in the new millennium if current trends continue. To date there has not been a break in the private sector coalition of health care. Managed care companies have not demanded government price controls on their for-profit brethren in the pharmaceutical companies, but that day may come.

The coming price war could take a number of forms. First, if a drug benefit is added to Medicare, then drug pricing will clearly become a policy issue particularly favored by democrats. Medicare has never fully flexed its purchasing muscle for prescription drugs, because drugs have not been a covered item under Medicare. (As we have discussed elsewhere, this also explains why the pharmaceutical industry has been opposed to drug coverage under Medicare: it fears that such coverage would lead to a national formulary or, worse yet, a national fee schedule for medications, as exists in Australia, France, and many other countries.) But there is a precedent for price controls in the United States. Under the Medicaid program, the federal government introduced best-price regulation to ensure that Medicaid programs would never have to pay a higher price than the rate offered to a large private sector bulk purchaser.

A second possible form of price war could take place because of the reinvigoration of the pharmacy benefit management (PBM) industry. By the early 1990s, PBMs claimed to have upwards of seventy-five million covered lives (although there may have been some double counting). As PBMs' apparent clout grew, they were quickly gobbled up by pharmaceutical companies under the mistaken belief that these organizations had tight control over patients, physicians, and the prescribing habits of those physicians. PBMs were never particularly successful at moving market share of medications around between competing companies; detailing and direct-to-consumer advertising were more effective. In actuality, PBMs were really no more than group purchasing vehicles and administrative processors rather than powerful controllers of pharmaceutical selection decisions.

PCS, one of the leading PBMs, bought for $4 billion in 1994 by pharmaceutical giant Eli Lilly, was sold to Rite-Aid in 1998 for $1.5 billion. Similarly, Smith-Kline Beacham sold off their PBM, Diversified Pharmaceutical Services, to Express Scripts for $700, less than a third of the purchase price five years earlier. These new super-PBMs, PCS Rite-Aid and DPS/Express Scripts, may be agents for turbocharging the PBM process, particularly if the employers or other managed care intermediaries who hire them back them up by enforcing generic and therapeutic substitution.

A third possibility is for the large HMOs to gang up on the pharmaceutical and medical technology industry. Imagine all the Blues plans acting as one big, mean pharmaceutical purchaser, or all the nonprofit HMOs that are members of the HMO Group (the consortium of large nonprofit HMOs) doing the same. What if the consolidation in health insurance continues? How much clout will Aetna U.S. Healthcare or Cigna have in the future?

Drug prices will become a very contentious issue in the next three years. Key in the debate will be consumers. The managed care industry's initial response to escalating drug costs has been to pass the burden onto the consumer in the form of higher copayments overall or through three-tiered formularies whereby consumers have to pay different levels of copays for different classes of drugs. For example, the *Wall Street Journal* reported that in Cigna's HMO the average cost of prescriptions increased by 44 percent from 1995 to 1998 at a time when health premiums rose only modestly. For brand-name drugs, Cigna's increase was 92 percent over the same period. These increases forced Cigna to increase consumers' copayment from a flat fee of $5 per prescription to up to $40 per prescription for the most costly medications. Aetna U.S. Healthcare reportedly planned to raise its copayment to $15 in 1999. Making the consumer aware of the price of prescription medication will encourage political pressure, particularly if the elderly are affected by these copayment increases. Even though long-term care represents the highest share of out-of-pocket costs on average for the elderly (approximately 42 percent of the elderly's out-of-pocket costs were for long-term care in 1996), this is a less common burden than out-of-pocket expenditure for medications (18 percent). Drug price wars will be bitter, and they may be political if the pharmaceutical industry maintains a "You can't touch us" stance.

The Case for Strategy Innovation

As we have discussed previously, we are witnessing a massive shift from defined benefit to defined contribution. This shift is going to shape the way in which consumers get health insurance, whether they are covered under Medicare or Medicaid or by their employers. This change is unlikely to reverse and is consistent with American values. In the face of this shift to defined contribution, a few very powerful but undifferentiated health plans will continually acquire each other and consolidate their positions. These are commoditized giants seemingly incapable of differentiating their service offering to the public. Increasingly, however, there *will* be differentiation—not at the level of the managed care plan but at the level of the care unit, be it a medical group or hospital or specific individual physician or group of physicians. Increasingly, consumers will become aware of the variation in clinical performance among these players. For example, Blue Shield of California's Access Plus HMO has conducted surveys of member satisfaction with specialty referrals, analyzing all of the different care units in California. Blue Shield found, within the same HMO, that satisfaction with specialty referrals varied from approximately 5 percent of patients saying they were "very satisfied" in one medical group to 95 percent in another. The variation within an HMO is much, much greater than the variation between HMOs, and that variation will eventually become more evident to consumers. Once consumers have the ability to differentiate, they may start doing much more voting with their feet, although it is not clear that the public will necessarily follow whatever the *Consumer Reports* of health care indicates as superior performance.

A big question for the managed care industry and for the provider community is, Will new products be created? Will new channels of distribution be created? Who will be the major innovators? Unfortunately, judging from the landscape, it is unlikely that the traditional managed care plans will be the source of innovation in health care. Rather, we are more likely to see new entrants who provide some fresh and new ideas in respect to the health care system. We are likely to see companies that use information technology as an entry point. Healtheon is the much-vaunted example of this strategy aimed at using the Internet to lubricate the administrative processes of managed care, particularly the linkage between physicians and health plans. It remains to be seen whether Healtheon can transform the field or whether it is simply a new technology applied to a dysfunctional set of relationships—paving the cow path.

The managed care industry has suffered financially and is unable to innovate in the medical management area. One place to look for innovation in the future, however, is to some of the traditional group and staff model HMOs—Kaiser, Henry Ford, and Harvard Pilgrim Health Care in particular. These plans have a dedication to the field, and they are committed to dealing with some of the central unresolved problems, namely developing effective medical management tools and the information infrastructure to support them. The field must look to Kaiser and other large nonprofit HMOs for some new ideas of how to fundamentally change health care delivery to improve quality and reduce costs, because it is unlikely that such innovation in care delivery will come from the commercial HMOs.

Kaiser and its sister HMOs are likely to be important innovators in the future, as they have been in the past. Similarly, others in the not-for-profit community have the luxury of avoiding the scrutiny of the marketplace. Blue Cross and Blue Shield plans, such as Blue Shield of California, could play important leadership and innovation roles in differentiating themselves from their for-profit competitors, which are significantly challenged by Wall Street's demands.

Will Wall Street be happy with for-profit providers? It seems unlikely that Wall Street will ever get back to being as euphoric as it once was about the potential in the health care area. Yes, health care is a big business, but analysts tend to get carried away with the large numbers. PPM companies rose to prominence partly because analysts got seduced with the simple arithmetic: if there's $200 billion of physician service money, 10 percent of it represents a market of $20 billion, no matter what *it* is. If margin could be created in the physician services area, then the sheer scale would make it an enormously exciting market opportunity. However, it's not nearly as easy as one might think to consolidate and add value in this business, because health care is such a local good. This is why one is critical of simply extrapolating the experience in other services to the health care system. Trying to find the McDonald's of health care underestimates the complexity of health care delivery and the way that health care delivery is integrated into local communities and into local patterns of practice. But if we can't use McDonald's as a model, where else do we look for innovation?

Medical care is practiced in a small space of possibility. Most of the actors in health care delivery are not innovating: they are just trying do the same things for less, and they are not happy about it. Even the entrepreneurial market innovators have stalled in health care delivery, and the relentless march of technology, particularly pharmaceuticals, is putting more pressure on a strained system, not less. We need to break out of the box in our strategies for health care organizations of all types. We need new business models. We need to innovate.

Chapter Eleven

Leadership and White Space

The Struggle for Strategy Innovation in Health Care

Strategy innovation has stalled in health care. No one has really envisioned a radical new future for U.S. health care that combines compassion, caring, cure, and coherence. No one has really explored the "white space"—imagining a whole new approach to the future.

It's often said that health care is a rapidly changing business. Who are we kidding? Health care moves at glacial speed compared to most other industries. Hospitals, physicians, and drug companies get the same share of the money (give or take a percentage point or two) that they have for thirty years or more. Government, business, and households pay about the same share of the health care pie as they did in the late 1960s. Most of U.S. health care is paid for on a discounted fee-for-service basis. Most doctors still practice in twosies and threesies with little or no sophisticated information infrastructure to guide their clinical practice.

True, we have rearranged the deck chairs on the *Titanic*. Travelers, Metropolitan, Prudential, and a whole host of medium and small insurers are no longer in the health insurance game. True, we have had new entrants in the HMO business. True, we have seen some Blue Cross plans and community hospitals convert to for-profit status. True, we have seen experiments in health care

delivery come and go, but most of these—such as PPM companies—have been fads, not a fundamental redefinition of the field.
Health care reorganizes around the fringes and futzes with financing mechanisms, but it has avoided any form of deep change or
serious restructuring (particularly in health care delivery) compared to such industries as financial services, which have gone
through fundamental changes in the last twenty years.

Compare health care to high technology. Where is the
Microsoft, the Intel, the Sun, the Charles Schwab, the Yahoo!, the
amazon.com? Health care is a trillion-dollar industry, ten times the
size of the computer industry. Health care is larger than the whole
high-tech sector put together. Yet our spending on R&D in health
services is less than 1 percent of revenues (except for pharmaceuticals and medical technology at around 15 percent), which is pitiful compared to most other high-technology businesses, which
spend more than 7 percent of sales on R&D.

We are not serving consumers' need for health or health care.
Patients are voting with their feet by embracing alternative therapies and providers. Consumers pay some $28 billion out of pocket
for alternate therapies, which equals the out-of-pocket costs for
physician services. *Time* magazine reports that the number of visits to alternative therapy providers equals the number of visits to
family practitioners.

Gary Hamel and C. K. Prahalad are widely regarded as being
among the leading thinkers on strategy. In a nutshell, their argument *Competing for the Future* (1994) is that successful companies,
through foresight and the development of a strategic architecture
for change, redefine their industry and sometimes create whole
new ones. These companies are built not only to last but also to
pass competitors by exploring the unexplored white space.

Strategy as an Emergent Process

In a recent opinion article ("Strategy Innovation and the Quest for
Value," *Sloan Management Review,* 1998), Hamel describes strategy
innovation as an emergent process. Drawing on complexity theory,
he argues that order arises from simple, deep rules. According to
Hamel, strategy emerges when the following preconditions are met:

- *New voices.* Hamel writes, "Bringing new genetic material into the strategy process always helps to illuminate unconventional strategies." Diversity, youth, and attitude enable successful strategy innovation.
- *New conversations.* Create dialogue across organizational and industry boundaries.
- *New passions.* "Harness the power of purpose," as William Pollard, chairman of ServiceMaster, has put it. Unleashing passion is key to innovation in strategy and, we might add, to effective execution of strategy.
- *New perspectives.* Create what Hamel terms "new conceptual lenses that allow individuals to reconceive their industry."
- *New experiments.* Launch a series of small, low-risk experiments in the marketplace and learn from the results.

How does health care stack up? In health care we have a long way to go to create organizations with true innovation in strategy. Using Hamel's analysis of the preconditions of innovation provides some clues:

- *Old voices.* Health care hears old voices. We are drowning in intransigent conservative stakeholders like the AMA, which fires its editor because he publishes evidence that shines light on a contemporary public policy debate. We have a narrow view of health as a by-product of medical care instead of as the result of a broad set of social and economic determinants. We lack diversity in leadership and management, in terms not only of race and gender but also of age and background.
- *Old conversations.* We are still fighting ideological battles from another age: single payer versus managed competition, capitation versus fee for service. Leaders in academic medicine talk in hushed tones about the Flexner report as if it came out last week.
- *Old passions.* The passion in health care has waned. Idealists raised on Medicare and Medicaid have become tired cynics. Pollyanna staffers from policy-wonk schools get the idealism beaten out of them after a few months of Let's Make a Deal policymaking in Congress and the state capitols. Aspiring hospital CEOs have to wait in line as a tired crew from the 1960s rotate jobs within the club.

• *Old perspectives.* Health care has few outside leaders and not much cross-fertilization from other industries. Where are the Jim Barksdales of health care, with career spells at AT&T, Federal Express, and Netscape? How do we see health care with a different lens if we are all using the same glasses? Little external perspective is brought to bear in health care because health care is an incredibly insular industry in terms of its leadership. Most health care leaders are products of the field, and there is not a good deal of exchange among the various elites even within the "360 of health care." Health care consultants tend to be industry obsessed, and health care policy wonks don't get out much. We end up breathing our own exhaust.

• *Old experiments.* We fall prey to fads. We never fully implement experiments. We don't learn from mistakes. We don't try, test, and modify as well as we should.

Why Health and Health Care Are Different

In fairness, health care is huge and complicated. It is not just a business but an important social service. It is a cottage industry of professionals. It has significant government involvement. It is deeply personal. All these factors make strategy innovation more difficult. But they do not excuse us from trying.

Asymmetry of information between the user and provider of health services differentiates health care from other forms of goods and services. The health economics literature points out that physicians are required to act as agents for the patient. When you buy a physician service, you have to give up a certain amount of autonomy simply because it is impossible to arm yourself with as much information, knowledge, training, and experience as the doctor. But in the world of the Internet, many consumers believe they can become as knowledgeable as the physician. In fact, the old proverb "a little knowledge is a dangerous thing" is probably true. Physicians get frustrated that they are dealing with more sophisticated customer-patients who come to them armed with Internet printouts and an in-your-face attitude. But these patients' questions and information base are not necessarily always better. In some cases they are worse, and a good deal of the interaction that could have been spent productively dealing with the patient's problems is instead spent screwing around, sorting through a bad bibliography drawn from unscientific sources. Yet no matter how dysfunctional this approach, more and more consumers are doing it because the health care system is failing them.

Health and illness are very personal, intimate, and potentially frightening. Health care and healing have serious spiritual and cultural dimensions. The relationship you have with your physician is not quite the same as your relationships with other knowledge professionals, such as lawyers and accountants. You may lose sleep over the interaction with your lawyer or your accountant, but it's not going to kill you. The ideal relationship with your physician, particularly as you reach the age of morbidity, is much deeper and much more personal. But the system is failing to deliver healing and compassion. Organs and body functions are restored while the whole patient is ignored. The system is failing to serve.

Lessons from Other Industries

The Pace of Change: Internet Time or Glacial Erosion?

We can learn from other industries, such as financial services, that are going through rapid and profound transformation. Banking and insurance giants are consolidating, and explosive innovators are transforming the field. We can learn from other industries about the speed at which organizational change can come about. For example, in 1996 Charles Schwab conducted less than one-third of its trading volume on-line. Within twenty-four months, two-thirds of its transactions were on-line.

In U.S. health care it's taken thirty years to get to a point where 15 percent of reimbursement is under anything but the traditional fee-for-service system. Even the penetration of on-line claim submissions has been a slow and laborious process over the last twenty-five years. Most managed care is in preferred provider organizations (PPOs) or point of service (POS), a small step from indemnity. There is tremendous resistance in this industry to structural change, partly because of the natural conservatism of the institutions.

Hospitals and physicians have organizational time clocks that are geared more to geological speed than to Internet speed, and their institutions change very slowly. The rhetoric of the field is one of rapid structural change, but to observers outside the industry, change is taking place at a pace akin to that of glacial erosion. There are certainly some new names, but the behavior of the actors is really not that different. U.S. medical care is still largely fee for service. The major innovation that occurred in the last twenty years probably was the DRG, which provided further incentives to move care out of the hospital.

Information Infrastructure as Platform for Innovation

A second key lesson we can learn from other industries is the potential payoff from investing in information infrastructure. There has been enormous investment in the financial services industry, and upwards of 10 percent of revenues has been applied to information infrastructure. This in turn has enabled a massive transformation in the institutions—the brands, the services—a transformation that pervades all aspects of our lives. It's not just that Charles Schwab can give you quotes on-line or that you can buy and sell stocks but that the infrastructure for money globally and locally is greatly changed from the past. The kinds of instruments that were once available only to the Rockefellers are now available to the middle class. The average consumer holds his or her assets in stocks rather than banks. Consumers can withdraw cash anywhere in the world using a plastic card. These radical alterations in the field are a function of new visions coupled to investment in the information infrastructure.

In health care we have not made those massive investments. Health spending on information technology has increased from approximately 1 percent of revenues to 3 percent of revenues, but it is still largely focused on automating internal hospital care processes or the insurance function. We still have a pathetically low penetration of clinical information systems in the hands of doctors. The electronic medical record is a permanently emerging technology, one that has been just over the horizon for the last thirty years despite some very important breakthroughs technologically and culturally. Despite the progress that has been made, the serious work that has been done by pioneers, and the millions of venture capital dollars that have flowed into this field, we still don't see computers in the hands of doctors. They may have them for their 401(k) plans, but they don't have them for their day-to-day clinical needs.

Skeptics point to the fact that medicine is a mobile profession and therefore not a very easy target to automate. What doctors do is complicated and legitimately idiosyncratic, they claim. The kinds of choices doctors have to make don't tend to be as clear-cut, simple, and programmable as the kinds of mechanistic decision making or actions that many other jobs and professions have.

All that may be true, but there is considerable potential still to be tapped related to the use of electronic infrastructure in administration and clinical applications, particularly in the physician's office. The potential of new technology is one of the few positive signs on the horizon that allow us to imagine a health care system that is both cheaper and better. Imaginatively applied, information technology could provide an enormous breakthrough in both productivity and performance.

Standardization and Customization

A third learning from other industries is the value of standardization as a step to mass customization. By developing standards, whole industries can take off; for example, MS-DOS, Windows, hypertext markup language (HTML), Intel processors, Java, and Postscript each in its own way spurred growth of information technology. Through standardization, quality can be improved, and whole new products can be invented to customize service offerings on those standard platforms.

Medical care in the United States is characterized by enormous variability in utilization. The *Dartmouth Atlas of Health Care,* developed by Dartmouth University and the AHA, has brought to the public Dr. Jack Wennberg's pioneering work demonstrating the enormous variation in utilization of medical services among different neighboring communities. In many instances this was explained by the density of distribution of physician resources and beds—the *Field of Dreams* effect: if you build it, they will come. But the atlas also demonstrated the vagaries of medical practice and the degree to which there could be three-, four-, five-, even tenfold variations in the use of various services, depending on the community in which the patients happened to reside.

There have been significant innovations in measurement of health care quality, a first step in limiting inappropriate variation. For example, the Center for Healthcare Improvement (Dr. Don Berwick's group in Boston), the National Committee on Quality Assurance, and the Foundation for Accountability, among others, have all made contributions to improving the measurement and management of quality. But we still have enormous variation in health care, and we are not much closer to transparency of performance metrics.

Increasingly we will see the creation and release of very fine grain information on physicians—batting averages, if you like—measured by procedure, by setting, by any other variable that you want. Physicians will balk at the release of such information. They will use the yeah-but defense. "Yeah, but have you adjusted for severity?" "Yeah, but have you adjusted for this, that, and the next thing?" They will be incensed, but the spread of this kind of information is part of the broader shift toward accountability and may, in its own way, lead to more standardization in the way in which clinical practices are carried out. By standardizing the component parts, health plans and other "care bundlers" yet to emerge can customize service offerings to suit consumers.

The Role of Market Leaders

The final key lesson one can draw from other industries is the importance of market leadership and market leaders in shaping the future of the industry. Hamel's work points to the breakthrough role played by companies that can imagine how whole industries can be transformed. Leaders create whole new industries—for example, Applied Materials in the semiconductor manufacturing equipment business or Charles Schwab in the discount financial services business. Leaders imagine places that the customer, the product, and their industry could go, and they conceive whole new business models and the strategies to get there.

Health care has had in its past some real market leaders. Kaiser Permanente presented a bold alternative vision for U.S. health care delivery. They can do so again. Overall, however, the voice of market leadership has been dampened in health care by the failure of undisciplined market leaders. Many of the for-profit market leaders (at least the market innovators) have stumbled badly in the last five years: Oxford Health Plans in managed care; for-profit hospital consolidators, such as Columbia/HCA; and drug companies that owned pharmacy benefit management companies—PBMs such as Prescription Card Service (Lilly) and Diversified Pharmaceutical Services (SmithKline Beacham). As we have discussed, the most spectacular rise and fall has been in the PPM sector, with Coastal Physicians, Phycor, FPA, and MedPartners taking their investors and employees on a rollercoaster ride of high drama, if not outright terror.

There is no Microsoft in health care. There is no General Electric. What we see instead are a series of relatively small, insular organizations that through arbitrage find a place in the sun for a brief moment, make a bunch of money, and then either blow up or leave. The industry is crying out for new business models, for new leaders, and for some of its traditional leaders, such as Kaiser, to reassert a very clear market superiority through innovation and measurable performance improvement.

Reconceiving the White Space: Where to Look for Innovation

Don't try to predict, try to imagine a better future. Combine the power of new information technology, the needs and wants of sophisticated consumers, and a broader definition of what creates health to imagine a better future. Among the many possible zones of innovation, three stand out:

- Applying our understanding of the determinants of health
- Designing health plans of the future
- Conceiving new reimbursement schemes for physicians

Determinants of Health

As discussed in Chapter Four, what creates health has very little to do with medical care and a lot to do with income, education, housing, socioeconomic status, and broader societal factors, such as the equality of income distribution. We can take this understanding of what creates health and apply it in our health policy, in our managed care plans, and in our communities. For example, in Vancouver, Canada, the Vancouver/Richmond Health Board (a recently created health authority organized to provide hospital health and community services across the continuum of care) announced that it was going to buy two low-income hotels and refurbish them for homeless, mentally ill, and indigent patients. The board recognized that many of its emergency room patients had medical problems associated with housing conditions. Although this sort of intervention might be a stretch for a for-profit health plan, is it such a stretch for a religiously based integrated system or a local county health department? Similar interventions are possible in such areas as substance abuse and mental health, domestic violence prevention, and transportation and social support for the chronically ill. We just need to broaden our vision. The next time a hospital board wants to buy a new MRI machine, let it buy twelve minivans instead. Use the vans to take poor people to medical appointments or to work. Improving their economic opportunities will improve their health status. If we are serious about improving the health of communities, we need to expand the vision.

Health Plans of the Future

The successful health plan of the future will not be simply a virtual single payer, a big mother of a purchaser that buys hospital and physician services in bulk and retails them back to employers. If that's all they do, they will eventually be replaced by business coalitions, private sector health insurance purchasing cooperatives (HIPCs), or Costco. Health plans could redefine themselves as mass customizers of health services. By developing standardized component parts of high quality, and core platforms that can be customized by consumers, a health plan could be a Dell or Gateway. Blue Shield of California's www.mylifepath.com is an early example of a mass customization strategy.

Physician Reimbursement

Capitation has stalled. Capitation was (and is) an interesting innovation when applied to large, sophisticated groups, because it provided an incentive for those groups to rethink how they could deliver health and health care. In theory, capitation was good because doctors could allocate the budget to maximize clinical outcomes. But like most budgeted systems, the people up the food chain ground down the budget and kept the payoff from any efficiencies. Similarly, physician groups, even the most sophisticated, struggled to find ways to manage, motivate, and reward individual physicians in the group so that they were simultaneously hard working, productive, parsimonious, and responsive to patients. Many groups resorted to splitting up the capitation payment using a discounted fee-for-service method.

To many doctors, capitation is the medical equivalent of tobacco farming: you are paid not to do something you want to do. Physicians like seeing patients and being paid for the transaction. Their work ethic dictates that they should be paid proportionally to their knowledge and time expended. (They would make lousy investment bankers.) That is why fee for service was so inherently appealing to physicians (especially when they can set their own prices).

How to Reinvigorate Health Care Strategy Innovation

If health care is to innovate like other industries, we need to reinvigorate the process of strategy making, as Hamel suggests. Specifically, we should try the following approaches:

- *Take a walk . . . off campus.* Most health care leaders and their entire organizations need to take a walk off campus. Look around and learn. Spend a day with a board member from another industry. Go to lunch with the most successful entrepreneur under thirty in your town. Read *Wired.* Go to a conference where thinkers from outside the health care industry reflect on the process and direction of change.

- *Make connections.* Innovation comes from connections among seemingly disparate ideas. In health care we need to connect with other trends in business. We need to see the rapid evolution of the new economy and learn from it.

- *Create Second Curve portfolios.* The Second Curve is the new business or the new way of doing business that is radically different from the old First Curve. We need to build a series of experiments that are designed to be edgy. Try them out, give them your best shot, expect them to fail, and learn from those failures.

- *Design innovation ecosystems.* Innovation in strategy is an emergent process. You must create an environment in which it can emerge. Is your strategy-making process engaging the smart young crazies in your organization? Do you have any smart young crazies? What would attract new thinking to your organization?
- *Develop metaphor factories.* A key tool in strategy innovation is the use of metaphors. Create metaphor factories where you systematically search for metaphors of how your industry could be completely reinvented.
- *Try viral marketing.* Tim Draper, a leading Internet venture capitalist, has popularized the term *viral marketing.* Many of his start-ups—including Hotmail, which was sold to Microsoft for $500 million—were based on the concept of viral marketing: give it away to build market dominance, and the money will follow. Hotmail collected fifteen million mail users in less than two years without spending more than $500,000 on marketing to get the first twelve million users. The business grew through viral marketing just like in the old Clairol commercial: "You tell two friends, and they tell two friends, and so on, and so on, and so on." The Internet is a powerful exponential communication media, and viral marketing has been enormously successful in building dominant brands on the Net.
- *Use humor, irony, and paradox.* Humor makes people think. Jokes are at their best when they reveal a fundamental truth. Most humor is derived from irony or paradox, the juxtaposition of the unrelated. Humor builds connections that can be leveraged to build insight and innovation. It's also easier to take a risk if you don't take yourself too seriously.

White Space in Health Care

Imagine innovations in strategy both large and small:
- *VISA Care.* A health plan and a bank give away VISA cards to uninsured bank customers that allow those customers to access any network physician at the health plan rate. There is no underwriting because there is no coverage (coverage could be an experience-rated option). By mailing the cards to all uninsured customers, the health plan adds to its purchasing power and clout with providers. The bank expands its cardholder base. The cus-

tomer benefits from the health plan pricing and may not postpone needed visits out of fear of price gouging.

- *Real group practice.* Alternative therapists, internists, chiro-practors, manicurists, massage therapists—all under one roof. Imagine real groups of health, healing, and caring professionals to care for the whole person.
- *E-Bay medicine.* E-Bay is the mother of all electronic flea markets, a place where buyers and sellers can meet in cyberspace. Hospitals have spare capacity, and physicians are oversupplied in the community. Need an appointment tomorrow at 9:00 with a dermatologist? Where is the E-Bay of health care, the electronic flea market to recycle excess capacity?
- *Disney and AOL do healthutainment.* Health promotion and disease prevention are about behavior modification. Imagine entertainment-based health care where everything from video games to soaps to sitcoms to chat rooms to electronic agents reinforce highly personalized behavior modification messages. Imagine being brainwashed to health by your own personal Big Brother.

The Leadership Dimension

Leaders play a key role in strategy innovation, but they do not have to do it all themselves. Rather, they need to create the environment for innovation in strategy. Too many CEOs are stuck on the vision thing. They perceive themselves as failures if they do not single-handedly conceive the new and different future. If the truth be known, that kind of thinking may be an impediment to innovation in strategy. Better to build an ecosystem in which strategy innovation can flourish than to single-handedly create the product.

Health care is ripe for change. If we don't do it, someone else might.

Chapter Twelve

Health Care in the New Millennium

The Long Boom Meets the Civil Society

The future is more popular than ever. Fueled by the coming of the new millennium, by dazzling new technologies, and by the roller-coaster of the global market, interest about where we are headed in the long run is at an all-time high. It is a good time for prognostication and prediction. But the dirty little secret of futurism is that we cannot predict the future. Serious scientists have tried (from the inventors of the Delphi technique to chaos theorists), but perfect prediction remains elusive. That doesn't mean there is no value in thinking systematically about the future. On the contrary, if you don't think systematically about the future, you run the risk of not participating in it.

Peter Schwartz and Daniel Yankelovich are two of the best thinkers about where we have been and where we are headed. As applied social scientists, they have guided corporate leaders and policymakers through their consulting, speaking, and writing.

In "The Long Boom" (an article in *Wired*) Peter Schwartz, who literally wrote the book on scenario planning, goes a little further than simply portraying a range of scenarios that describe the underlying uncertainty ahead. Instead, "The Long Boom" is a single scenario, a call to action, and a radically positive view of what is possible in the future. Openness (in many arenas, from global trade to culture to organizational forms to computer architecture), new technology, and the growth in Asia combine to create the Long Boom, a period of economic growth and prosperity that lasts a quarter-century. A rising tsunami lifts all boats.

"The Long Boom" is a refreshing, in-your-face view of what could happen if we do things right. CEOs love it; it lets them sleep well at night, knowing that all that money they are making is serving some broader positive purpose. Some find the utopian, techno-possibilist tone a little too Pollyannaish.

Dan Yankelovich's book *Dialogue* (1998) does take some exception to the Long Boom concept. Yankelovich has spent an entire illustrious career taking the pulse of the United States and counseling U.S. leaders on where to head next. In *Dialogue* he cites "The Long Boom" as a good example of the boosterist free-market vision for the world and argues persuasively for greater dialogue between this vision of the future and the vision of the Civil Society in which "the market has a place, the market in its place." Yankelovich sees a battle for the soul of the American public: Are we only driven by the market, or are we also driven by a higher set of values of family, community, and civil behavior?

I violently agree with both Schwartz and Yankelovich. We need more optimism about what is positive about the future. The Long Boom concept sets an agenda for opening trade, encouraging innovation, and using new technology for the broader social good. It is unashamedly upbeat, and lord knows we need some kind of positive spin on the future.

But I also agree with Yankelovich that the market doesn't have a conscience. Absent thoughtful intervention by government and the independent sector, not only will the market fail to work very well, but our society will become uncivilized. Yankelovich emphasizes the role of politics and democratic institutions in shaping the Civil Society and tries to galvanize his readers to engage in meaningful dialogue about the future and not simply let the market sweep over them. He sees more of the negatives of the new economy: crime, moral decay, political apathy, selfishness and mean spiritedness in our debates, and urges for a more balanced view of the future. Yankelovich asks this basic question: What do we stand for as a society?

Four Scenarios for Health Care

We can use the Long Boom and the Civil Society as constructs for creating a new set of scenarios more tailored to a health care audience. Scenarios ought to represent the range of uncertainty in the future. The Long Boom is one scenario for the global business environment. Further scenarios need to be constructed to help decision makers identify threats and opportunities that demand a planned response. Scenarios can be particularly helpful in framing what I term *long-tailed decisions* (those decisions taken today that have long-term consequences, such as investing in pharmaceutical R&D, building a $200 million acute-care facility, or doubling the size of medical schools). The other cardinal rule of scenario planning is that the scenarios should be tailored to the user. The Long Boom and the Civil Society are about the environment in general, not the health care system. But the Long Boom and the Civil Society represent possible dimensions of uncertainty, a space that can be filled with scenarios specific to health care.

On one dimension, civility, our society can become less civilized, or it can move toward the opposite end of the continuum to the Civil Society, in which decency, values, and orderly debate ensue. On the second dimension we have the Long Boom versus the Short Boom. The Short Boom suggests that the current economic expansion is merely part of the business cycle and that the underlying pattern of long-term growth in the U.S. economy remains relatively constant over the next twenty years, as it has in the last: 2.7 percent real growth. The Short Boom implies we are overdue for a recession.

Using these two dimensions to define the range of uncertainty, we can create four scenarios for health care, as illustrated in Figure 12.1: Community Care, Medicare Choice for All, Ugly Recession, and Adam Smith Beats Karl Marx—Health Care as Financial Services.

Scenario 1: Community Care

This is a Civilized Recession, if there is such a thing. As the Asian flu turns to major emerging-market pneumonia, the bloom is off the global rose. It becomes apparent that emerging markets were

Figure 12.1. Four Scenarios for Health Care.

	Short Boom	Long Boom
Civil Society	Community Care	Medicare Choice for All
Uncivil Society	Ugly Recession	Adam Smith Beats Karl Marx— Health Care as Financial Services

not fueling much of U.S. corporate profits in the 1990s in the absolute but that those markets were fueling a good deal of the *growth* in profits. Asia and the emerging markets of Eastern Europe and Latin America remain committed to a market path, but the restructuring needed is serious, painful, and long term. The financial bailouts put a strain on the United States as global banker, and the economy gets dragged down with the burden. The technology sector takes the biggest hit as the Asian slowdown meets a falloff in domestic demand for technology. Everyone is on the Net, and no one knows why. It becomes clear that the continuous upgrading of computers in the mid-1990s was a pointless quest for faster Web surfing. Sure the Net is part of the culture; sure many companies use it as a channel for communication and transactions; but it is only one channel of many. The great technology infrastructure boom is largely complete in 1999: virtually every family with household income over $50,000 has a computer, and less well off households never really take to the Net computer. As a result, rates of growth in the computer industry moderate substantially early in the new millennium.

Congress remains committed to a balanced budget despite leaner times, which has meant that some programs have had to be cut. But the legacy of the Clinton administration is a balanced budget *and* a more flexible and responsive federal bureaucracy. The national debates on welfare and Social Security of the late 1990s took advantage of the years of prosperity and put in place sustainable funding for major federal social programs. But most important, the new federalism requires and encourages much more self-reliance for communities to govern their own affairs. Cities and regions are increasingly responsible for shaping their own future.

America is focusing on building its local communities. Fiscal conservatism and social liberalism, which were so hard to reconcile at the national level, are implemented most effectively at the local level. Problems of education, race relations, homelessness, and health care all seem less daunting when resolved locally. Health care is the big surprise. In the early years of the Clinton administration, health care seemed destined for reform by the federal government. In the mid-1990s it was the market that reformed the system. But the managed care backlash kept building until the debate of 2000, when tight federal regulation of the managed care industry was rejected by Congress in favor of guidelines and incentives for those institutions that demonstrated quality care to local communities.

Innovation starts, not in the biggest cities, but in such places as Portland, Orlando, Des Moines, and Kansas City. Here the leaders of nonprofit health care institutions are instrumental in fashioning the new community compromise. Following the pioneering lead of a select few, community after community develops effective dialogue among managed care plans, hospitals, physicians, employers, and local government. In many cases, the fact that only two or three health plans dominate the market is instrumental in bringing them to the community table. But the key catalytic role is played by local hospitals, physicians, and community business leaders who developed coalitions focused on making their communities healthier. Health care is often the number one employer, so it is in everyone's interest to see that it thrives, especially in a recession, when unemployment in the globally competitive markets (such as manufacturing) is on the rise.

Local and state governments are willing partners in community-based reform. The balanced budget mentality coupled to economic downturn means it can't be business as usual for state and local government. Shoring up the safety net with categorical program funding, disproportionate share money (DSH), and FFS Medicaid is simply not feasible. The safety net would be overwhelmed as the number of eligible people rises in the recession. Instead, local governments increasingly seek federal and state waivers to develop collaborative public-private programs. In most cases the waivers involve Medicaid. In addition, provider-sponsored networks (PSNs) become popular under Medicare, particularly those run by large nonprofit provider groups that hire savvy marketers and insurance executives to help position the local, nonprofit PSN as a kinder, gentler alternative to money-grubbing commercial HMOs.

There is a lot of experimentation, much of it funded by private foundations. Some communities are more successful than others, which is perhaps the most troubling issue. The quality of health care and health in communities varies substantially across the country.

Scenario 2: Medicare Choice for All

The Long Boom continues. Asia bites the bullet and deals with the bloated bureaucracies and shaky lending practices that got it into trouble. The basic engine remains intact: huge populations who want a better life and are committed to the global market as a means of achieving it. The United States rises to the occasion to enable Asia and the other emerging markets to thrive. As banker, statesman, and business partner, the United States plays a leadership role in supporting balanced economic development in Asia by fostering markets *and* democracy.

Low interest rates, the movement of baby boomers from being net debtors to net savers, and continued competitive pressure to raise productivity through technological and organizational innovation combine to fuel an investment boom that lasts through the first decade of the new millennium. New technologies, from computers to biotechnology, create the economic base for the future. The Clinton administration's decision to double the NIH budget unleashes a wave of new innovation in a variety of industries, not just health care.

As more baby boomers turn fifty, the triple whammy looms: aging parents needing long-term care, kids still in college or at home in their late twenties, and continued corporate restructuring to meet a rapidly changing global marketplace. The underlying sense of individual social insecurity despite overall economic prosperity prompts a national debate on the New Safety Net. The New Safety Net debate is not so much about the old and the poor but about social programs relevant for the new economy. In particular, the debate centers on the needs of the vulnerable middle class who are one job change away from losing health benefits; who need portability in pension, life, and disability insurance; and who might become unemployed ten years shy of eligibility for Medicare and Social Security. By 2005, the top five employers in the United States are organizations that were once called temporary help companies. Each of them issues over two million W-2s every year. Millions of successful working people are free agents—solo practitioners in their home-based offices. But health care remains a big cost and a key vulnerability for them. The time is right for change.

Medicare risk is one model of public-private reform. After an inconspicuous start in 1986, Medicare risk took off in the late 1980s and early 1990s. The program grew rapidly to enroll 16 percent of the Medicare population by 1998. Then PSNs were developed, but nobody came to the party. The institutions most eager to participate as PSNs were the ones least qualified to do it. Eight gynecologists set up a Medicare PSN in Alabama and failed miserably, both clinically and economically. The widespread failure of PSNs in the late 1990s spawns a wholesale review of Medicare as part of the new president's Millennial Commission. The commission fixes Medicare by developing an orderly transfer from fee for service to a competitive managed care model. Three key reforms take place:

• Risk adjustment is enacted to ensure that HMOs and qualified PSNs are given incentives to manage care and not just dodge risk. The political and technical battles in getting a workable system of risk adjustment are substantial, but everyone recognizes that risk adjustment is critical if managed care is to move forward.

• Rigorous quality reviews are introduced that include accreditation and performance measurement of clinical outcomes and customer satisfaction. These federal standards are administered by two independent, nonprofit organizations—JCAHO and NCQA—on a deemed status basis. Quality assessment has become much more sophisticated with the maturing of the information infrastructure for capturing and analyzing clinical data and Medicare's mandating of certain data-collection standards.

• The opt-out provision in Medicare risk is modified to require the elderly to select health plans for a year at a time, albeit with the right to opt out of network for a higher copayment and deductible structure.

These reforms bring the Medicare+Choice model closer to the idealized vision of managed competition. The results are impressive. By 2005, 50 percent of the elderly are in Medicare+Choice programs. Prompted by the reforms, providers have significantly innovated in the management of chronically sick elderly patients. Hospitals and health systems, specialty carve-out organizations, and the brand-name health plans are virtually integrated to deliver seamless care to the elderly. Overall, analysts judge Medicare Choice to be better for the well, better for the sick, and better for the system.

Medicare Choice reform and the New Safety Net come together as the central debate issue of the 2006 congressional election. It becomes clear that Medicare and Social Security are unworkable programs for the baby boom bolus that will overwhelm the system in 2010 and beyond. Social Security is saved as an individual benefit paid for in real time by a working population taxed at a level high enough to sustain the needs of current recipients. Medicare cannot also continue operating on that basis. The pressure to broaden the funding base for Medicare and the need to provide the New Safety Net lead to sweeping reform. Every individual American is mandated to purchase health insurance. He or she can buy it through the Federal Medicare Risk Program at an actuarially adjusted rate; through any other qualified channel, such as large private sector employers, professional employment organizations (PEOs), and total benefits outsourcers (TBOs); or through public or privately sponsored health insurance purchasing cooperatives (HIPCs). Health benefits are now deductible as an individual tax benefit at half the basic rate of tax. Health benefits are no longer a deductible employee benefit for employers; as a result, most employers withdraw from health benefits administration. A basic Medicare Choice benefit is standardized, but HMOs and other managed care models compete fiercely with benefit wraparounds and styles of customer service.

The American public has come to terms with managed care and with the fact that it can never have security without a federal mandate that every American participates on an equal footing. The opponents of the legislation who tried to characterize it as big government are shouted down by the managed care industry, by providers, and by the vulnerable middle class. Most important, proponents of the bill could point to the success of the reforms in Medicare Choice. This time Americans aren't being asked to buy a car they haven't driven.

Scenario 3: Ugly Recession

We all knew it had to end sometime, but no one expected this. The Asian flu; the slow, ugly demise of the Clinton administration; and the end of corporate earnings growth bring the greatest postwar period of economic expansion to an end. The 1990s expansion covered up the truth of the new economy: despite overall economic expansion, most families in the United States are so over-leveraged in terms of time and money that they are one paycheck away from oblivion. As the stock market slumps backwards and the jobless numbers rise, more and more families are underwater. Car loans that exceed the value of the car, huge credit card debts, unpaid health care bills, and low or no growth in real wages for those who have jobs—all are typical. Everybody is worried about their own troubles.

The 2000 election turnout is the lowest ever. The legacy of the Clinton scandals is that the pressure of public scrutiny keeps good candidates away, and, worse yet, public apathy increases toward politics in general and Washington in particular. The new crop of political candidates are antiseptically clean, boring, and dull. The Republican president is elected as a "compassionate conservative," but there is no clear vision of what that means or how it will be translated into policy. The best interpretation is that compassionate conservative means, "I'm really sorry I'm cutting your entitlement program." This is a society that is hunkering down, everyone wrapped in his or her own little cocoon.

Welfare cuts at the height of the economic expansion become really painful as the recession deepens. States and local communities are not prepared fiscally or politically for the wave of new poor. A clear divide develops between those who are on the economic lifeboat and those who are off. The vast majority of working Americans breathe a sigh of relief because they are on the lifeboat, and although there is some sympathy for the less well off, no politician is galvanizing support to do anything about them.

Big cities are struggling with the health care issue. San Francisco, for example, rode high under the Clinton administration and Mayor Willie Brown, but now faces a "No Billy, no Willie" scenario. The city government, which embarked on a noble effort to create a universal coverage initiative in the city in 1998, finds itself in a battle to maintain its health care safety net. By 2004 it is in a fight to keep the jobs it created in the 1990s that are flying to low-cost states and countries, and it has to downsize city employees. The California safety net, which got by with over 20 percent uninsured during the height of the economic expansion, is devastated by the recession, and San Francisco is a prime example. It started with erosion of the numbers of healthy Medi-Cal patients to the private sector HMOs, leaving poor and chronically sick patients in the public sector. With the economic downturn, the uninsured and Medi-Cal rolls climbed just as state tax revenues dropped.

A Republican White House and Congress are united in balancing the budget through the recession. They preach responsibility and accountability. With tax revenues down and Social Security and defense inviolate, there is little wiggle room. DSH is cut deeply. Calls for the voluntary sector to serve the poor are widespread in Washington.

It is impossible for the news media to develop any sense of urgency about the rising numbers of uninsured. Already anesthetized to forty million uninsured, the public fails to become outraged that the number rises to sixty million in a three-year period. Like the proverbial frog that gets boiled one degree at a time without leaping out of the pot, the American public accepts that health care is not a right but a privilege to be enjoyed by the medically fortunate.

Politicians point to the transitory uninsured and insist that the vast majority who are both young and healthy will be covered by health insurance when the economy improves.

Health care is heavily tiered. There are some basket-case institutions kept afloat by bailing wire and the Robert Wood Johnson Foundation. The lucky employed have managed care coverage, but the managed care industry is full of uninspiring offerings that beat up doctors and hospitals on price and try to restrict access to services. The managed care industry, once the darling of Wall Street, has stalled badly in the late 1990s, and the smart money has left. HMOs and managed care are all there is, and neither the patients nor the doctors are particularly happy about it. Hospitals are struggling as the stock market sours: hospitals can no longer rely on investment income to shore up their weak operational results. For the lucky few, health care is very good; premiums are expensive and technology is extravagantly applied, but there are some who can afford it.

This is a selfish health care system; those who are doing OK don't complain. But no one in their right mind would say that it's the best we can do as a nation. Politicians won't touch it, Wall Street doesn't care about it anymore, and those in the game squabble over what there is—still a huge share of the American economy.

Scenario 4: Adam Smith Beats Karl Marx— Health Care as Financial Services

As the new millennium dawns, it becomes clear that the market is the dominant model for the planet. It varies enormously from the socialized markets of Scandinavia and the state-run markets of Asia to the mob-run markets of Russia. But the United States is the center of the universe, all-powerful, the source of innovation, and by far the wealthiest nation on earth. Market mechanisms help solve problems from pollution to education.

The three great pillars of globalization are Coca-Cola, CNN, and financial services. The United States has them all. But despite the name recognition for Coke and CNN, financial services is the leitmotif of the next millennium. The success of new financial instruments, the continuous upward move of the stock market, the application of new technology to serve consumers and investors— all encourage many industries to go the way of financial services.

For health care the lessons from financial services are taken to heart by employers, the managed care industry, providers, and consumers alike. Seven key changes take place:

• *The shift from defined benefit to defined contribution (DB to DC) is complete.* Just as pensions shifted from a defined-benefit format to a defined-contribution model in the 1980s, fueling the growth of 401(k) plans and mutual funds, so large employers and the federal government alike move health care from DB to DC. In Medicare, you have the right to trade up to a better Medicare plan with your own money. For the typical employee, health benefits come in the form of a monthly allowance to be applied to any number of health and wealth options, including traditional HMO-type products as well as plans that have restricted health coverage but expanded long-term care and disability coverage.

• *There is regulatory support for new products.* Just as Merrill Lynch helped shape the regulatory changes that enabled the creation of money market funds, so such innovators in financial services as Fidelity and Schwab start to take an interest in the health benefits market as a whole as a new source of funds flow. They push for regulatory changes that make health care operate more like other financial services, such as mutual funds and mortgages.

• *The health care value chain becomes like that of financial services.* In the mortgage banking business, regulatory changes and new product innovation in the 1980s radically transformed the value chain. In the old days, if you took out a mortgage with a bank, the bank sold it to you, it administered the repayment of the loan, and it kept the loan on its balance sheet. In the new world, the people who sell you the loan, bundle up like loans into standardized blocks that they resell to another party; meanwhile the processing and administration of the loan payments are done by a third party. You might even have used an independent mortgage broker to help you find the right loan. Similarly, with credit cards and mutual funds, the people who sell you the service don't necessarily underwrite the service or hold your money. These changes require three things: enabling legislation, intervening institutions to help markets function (such as Fannie Mae or the SEC), and entrepreneurial innovation enabled by new technology. In health care, new entities are created that separate the functions in the health care value chain. The people who sell you health insurance are different from those who bear the risk and are different from those who service you.

• *The federal government introduces risk rating and adjustment and creates Fannie Med.* Under pressure from the managed care and financial services industries, the federal government creates the Federal Medical Insurance Adjustment Board, known in the industry as Fannie Med. Its purpose is to act as a clearinghouse for health insurers and provider entities. Blocks of insured lives (like blocks of mortgages) are bundled and rebundled on a risk-adjusted basis by Fannie Med. The risk adjustment is very sophisticated. Inexpensive genetic screening tests are available and are used routinely in combination with traditional health risk appraisal methodologies to assess any individual's risk rating when he or she applies for health insurance. There are strict federal laws protecting the confidentiality of individuals' genetic information. Blocks of patients are genetically tested by Fannie Med, but individual data are kept confidential. Because all rates are bundled into community-standard blocks by Fannie Med, each insured life pays the same age-adjusted premium regardless of health status.

• *The consumer pays and chooses.* The individual consumer pays for the trade-up in health plan choice, but the base premium is paid for in a variety of ways, much as it was in the 1990s. Large employers orchestrate health benefits for their employees on a defined-contribution basis. But companies like Schwab and Fidelity are increasingly popular originators of health insurance because they package their offerings into interesting combinations—such as pension, long-term care, and health insurance accounts—with very simplified reporting. Similarly, credit card companies like VISA and American Express are extremely active in the market, offering managed care plans (so-called high-deductible HMOs) that are easy to administer for both patient and provider—with the swipe of a credit card. Products and channels proliferate because Fannie Med can reconcile the basic risk profile of the recipients with the costs of care provision. Horizontal specialists emerge, just as Countrywide did in the mortgage banking business in the mid-1990s as the key specialist in loans administration. But the principal benefit to consumers is choice; because they are risk-identified but community-rated at the source, they can sign up with any qualified provider group and change on a monthly basis with no fear.

• *Providers focus on risk-adjusted segments.* Providers are paid a risk-adjusted monthly payment based on the pool of members signed on in any given month. Because providers have no incentive to cherry-pick recipients, they can focus on those types of patients they want to serve: worried well, chronically ill, frequent users, sports nuts, diabetics, AIDS cases—the segments are endless. By 2010 there are three hundred thousand registered provider units in the United States, just about the same as the number of different mutual funds, and each has its own unique risk-adjusted focus and mission.

• *E-commerce provides the infrastructure.* The health care system borrows much of the e-commerce infrastrucure from financial services. A wide variety of e-health giants has emerged, including many financial service companies that migrate into health care, as well as health care–specific e-commerce companies. No one can remember how health care worked before the Internet.

Issues and Impacts

Scenarios are sketch maps of the future. They provide some clues about what may lie ahead. But their real value is to highlight the key issues—those threats and opportunities that demand a planned response. There are ten key issues that should be drawn from the scenarios I have just described.

1. *Vision.* The health care industry desperately needs a new vision. Managed competition among orderly vertically integrated systems wasn't such a bad idea, but we never implemented it. These scenarios represent alternate views of the environment for health care and some possible visions for the industry. If you don't like the future you see here—change it.

2. *Values.* We like to talk about values, and there are some pretty high-falutin' value statements out there in the health care industry. But judging from the evidence to date, we also have to

recognize that in health care we don't seem to value universality or equity. So what is it that we do value? Let's get clear about the values in health care and be honest. If we say we are a community-focused, not-for-profit hospital system dedicated to the health of our local community, then we should behave in such a way that those values are clearly detectable to human beings.

3. *Leadership.* Alan Hoops, CEO of PacifiCare, has wisely noted that the indemnity health insurance industry died too quickly, which caused HMOs to be unexpectedly thrust from being the opposition to being the mainstream. Hoops's point is that the managed care industry wasn't really prepared for the leadership role in health care, and they therefore have not performed as well as they should in public policymaking or in public relations. But if leadership and innovation don't come from the managed care industry, where else do we look? One place we ought to see more leadership is in the physician community. Doctors are clinically depressed. They don't feel they have control over their lives, and they are deeply vexed about the future. It is time for the medical profession to step up and describe a better future for health care, one that does not involve a return to 1973 or some other imagined golden age. In particular, they must attempt to deal with one of the most crucial questions: What should the future of specialty care be in the United States?

4. *Role of government in health.* Both the Long Boom and the Civil Society are anti–big government. But government—at federal, state, and local levels—is likely to have a big role in almost any scenario as payer, provider, regulator, and enabler. Of course we should look more closely at how government can be more effective in health care, but we cannot ignore the legitimacy of the government's role and its continued substantial financial presence. In particular, we should recognize that there is no such thing as voluntary universal coverage. If all Americans are to be covered, it will require some form of government mandate.

5. *The independent sector.* The independent sector of nonprofit community-based organizations, from the United Way to the Brookings Institution, plays a critical role in American life and in the concept of the Civil Society. Nowhere is that more true than in health care, where the nonprofit hospital sector still provides over

80 percent of the care. The independent sector needs to clarify its role in the health care system of the future. Is it a hypocritical bystander or the leader of meaningful change?

6. *Local versus national*. Health care is a local good, but we have a mix of national and local actors, both public and private. If health care is to be resolved as a local issue, will we tolerate the even larger regional disparities in health care that may result? Conversely, can a country as large, diverse, and politically challenged as the United States ever get it together to do a national program? In the private sector, where is the benefit of a national managed care presence? The leading HMOs in the country, Kaiser and United Healthcare, are far from national players. Kaiser still has 80 percent of its lives west of the Pecos, wherever that is; and United Healthcare has a tiny market share in such key managed care states as California and Arizona.

7. *Health policy and the new economy*. Neither the managed care industry nor Wonkworld has really come to terms with health care in the new economy. When an increasing share of the labor force is contingent, flexible, temporary, or free agents, where are the private products and public policies to serve the health care needs of the new economy and the new workforce?

8. *Innovation*. The health care industry is in desperate need of innovation across all its dimensions. We need innovation at the policy level in many areas, but particularly in the areas of risk adjustment, both in Medicare and in other insurance products, and of portability of health benefits. In the managed care industry, we need plans to develop new products that give consumers choice, low costs, and ease of use, without alienating the provider community. In health care delivery, we need clinical innovation in caring for the chronically ill in a cost-effective way. The list is endless. Other industries with high need for innovation invest significantly in R&D; with the exception of the pharmaceutical industry, health care generally spends nada on R&D, and it shows.

9. *New technology*. Much has been made of the information technology (IT) boom and the Internet as an agent of change, and there is much to be done in health care with the new tools of IT. In particular, e-commerce is likely to be a very important dimension of the future health care system; it will enable a more efficient form of pluralism. But of equal significance is the role of genomics

and genetic testing in the health care industry. The concept of experience-rated health insurance is seriously loony when genetic testing is widely available. These tools could be used for genetic redlining by nasty insurers who want to turbocharge cream skimming, or they could be the basis of a much more sophisticated form of risk adjustment for a whole generation of new products and policies.

10. *Consumers will be heard.* You cannot have a health care system in which benefit managers and health plan executives are deliriously happy, and patients and their doctors are angry and disappointed. The recent managed care backlash is testimony to that. But what is it that consumers want from health care? We will hear from consumers more and more, but the key problem will remain: consumers want anything, any time, any place, any way they want it, and they are not willing to pay much out of pocket to get it. Consumers are also voters, plan members, and patients. They want different things from their health care system at different times. Resolving the tension between these different roles will be a significant problem in any future.

Chapter Thirteen

| **Five Key Leadership Steps**

Health care is at a turning point. We can either keep going toward a default future where doctors are powerless and miserable in a world of discounted fee for service, like hamsters on a treadmill; where consumers scramble to get what they need and want from an unresponsive health care system; where health plans are commoditized giants with just enough incentive to stay in the game as low-margin players, unimaginative and unrewarded; and where the creators of new technology are frustrated that the fruits of the new science are unaffordable to many consumers who have to choose between leading-edge medical care and other necessities of daily living. We can envision a better future.

A Possible Future

The goal of this book has been to stimulate leaders to think about the long-term future of health care in the United States, not to present some preconceived solution. Leaders with vision will build consensus through debate and dialogue around values and principles.

Although the goal of the book is to stimulate others to think about the future, I have a private dream about how the U.S. health care system might evolve. A possible compromise is Medicare Choice for All, a system that achieves universal coverage by mandating that every citizen in the United States buy into the Medicare program, which would include a tiered drug benefit that provides drug coverage and a guaranteed base of long-term care coverage. Large employers could maintain separate experience-rated programs, but the tax treatment of health benefits would be uniform.

231

Half of the basic program cost would be deductible at the base rate of tax for individuals. This tax treatment of health benefits would require employers and their employees to give back some of the tax deductibility for health benefits that currently exists, estimated to be around $100 billion. The proposed policy would also provide a tax deduction as an incentive for individuals and the self-employed to purchase health insurance. Such a move would redistribute the tax subsidy from employers to small businesses and to individuals. The precise nature of this tax incentive would clearly depend on the fine-tuning of the floors and ceilings for Medicare. Clearly, the intent here would be to provide universal access to a program that has been pared down from its current form. It is a highly charged political question as to how low the floor could possibly be for Medicare recipients in terms of coverage.

The fixed floor of Medicare could be a base HMO plan with a restricted set of providers, or a basic fee-for-service plan with copayments and deductibles. Enrollees would trade up to get additional benefits, whether from managed care plans or from other forms of fee for service.

Involving all Americans in Medicare+Choice creates a number of important effects beyond the obvious one of universal coverage. First, it spreads the cost burden across the whole population. A full 80 percent of the uninsured are working people and their families; they would have an obligation to pay some toward their care. It also is clear that any universal scheme would have to involve significant subsidy for those in poverty. Second, such an approach removes the enormous cliff of the baby boom turning sixty-five. No other country has a health system in which people flip over from private coverage to public coverage at a certain age, which explains why countries like the United Kingdom, Sweden, and Germany have all experienced having much higher proportions of the population over sixty-five without their system collapsing. Third, the Medicare+Choice model and, alternatively, the Federal Employees Health Benefits model both preserve choice and allow for competition among insurers and health plans. Choice is an American value, even if it costs more money in the long run for the same benefit. Fourth, the politics of health care could be transformed if the system combined a sense of individual responsibility to pay for health insurance with a federal mandate to participate in the program, much in the way we are required to purchase auto insurance.

One important area of compromise in any proposed reform of Medicare or the health system as a whole will be around the issue of prescription drug coverage. It seems unlikely politically that any kind of national health program or an expansion of Medicare to cover prescription drugs could be secured if the pharmaceutical industry became the target of extreme price controls on the Canadian, French, or Australian models. The line in the sand for the pharmaceutical industry is likely to relate to a national formulary or any extreme form of price controls. The pharmaceutical industry's support could be secured for a program of coverage expansion provided that the program did not essentially want to regulate the pharmaceutical industry out of existence. The challenge is to design policy in which an innovative pharmaceutical industry can be preserved.

Further important elements of any broader expansion of Medicare Choice would involve encouraging the development of both the information infrastructure and the standards of quality in health care.

The notion of Medicare Choice for All is not a full-blown proposal but a sketch map for the future. The point here is not to propose a specific alternative but to suggest a compromise or to circumscribe the possible space in which a compromise consistent with prevailing American values might develop. The key challenge going forward is to have more of a dialogue about options for the future and to reinvigorate the national health debate. Meeting this challenge will require political leadership at state, local, and federal levels—a difficult task because it is so much easier to oppose than to propose in U.S. politics.

Five Key Leadership Steps

The Medicare Choice for All model is but one vision. Whatever vision of a better future we wish to follow, it will take leadership to get us there. There are five key leadership steps involved in creating any future for U.S. health care.

Step One: Agree on a Values Base

We will never make any progress toward universality in U.S. health care until we agree that there is no such thing as voluntary universal coverage. Similarly, we will not make any progress unless we agree that Americans fundamentally don't believe in equity. Progress toward universality will require an explicit recognition of floors and ceilings. What Americans really want is a floor below which no American falls and the right to trade up with their own money to a better waiting room with a better class of people.

Second, we need to agree that we are comfortable with risk adjustment instead of community rating. Again, the U.S. public will not tolerate cross subsidy once they have experienced a better deal on an experienced-rated basis. The belief in experience rating undermines the whole concept of community-rated insurance but nevertheless is fundamentally consistent with American values. To ensure that the health insurance system is operational and not totally dysfunctional requires methods of risk evaluation and risk adjustment to compensate providers, health plans, and others for the fact that the burden of disease is very asymmetrically distributed. If we are not going to community-rate, then we must risk-adjust to avoid what are fundamentally extremely harmful selection effects that can wreak economic havoc on the health care financing system and on health care delivery.

Third, we need national minimum standards but local responsiveness and accountability. America will not tolerate a one-system, federal, standardized health care delivery system. There is huge variation, and it needs to be reduced, but this reduction is unlikely to occur through federal government mandate. Indeed, if one looks at other standardized universal systems, such as Australia, Canada, Italy, and France, one sees tremendous local variation (albeit in a national framework), not so much in the pattern of care, which is a universally variable phenomenon, but in terms of local governance issues. In no large country is health a nationally mandated, nationally administered, nationally standardized activity, either in its financing or regulation.

Fourth, we must understand the system of health. We need a societal debate on a broader vision of health, one that builds on a greater understanding of the determinants of health and provides a clearer conception of what constitutes appropriate health care delivery. Foundations, academics, and the media can play an important role in educating the public and the provider communities about what really causes improvements in health status—even though the public and providers may not like the results, because the interventions may indeed smell too much like socialism for the average American to tolerate. It is important to fully understand what really does create and constitute health.

Fifth, we must recognize the legitimacy of the roles played by the market, the government, and the independent sector. One cannot conceive of a U.S. health care system run by the market exclusively, nor can one conceive of a system in which the market doesn't participate. Similarly, government has a large and increasing role in health care, as does the independent sector. None of these sectors is likely to disappear.

The proportion of health care paid by the three key actors—government, households, and employers—has remained relatively constant for thirty years, since the enactment of Medicare. The big question for the future is, Does the private sector contribution have to flow through the employers? It is in how we answer this question that we have the biggest potential for change, because the health system of the future may get further and further away from being tied to the employment base. Most Americans don't work for large corporations, and there is therefore a huge opportunity to disconnect health coverage from employment, or at least from working for specific employers. Much more workable would be a system in which health care coverage is tied to employment on a payroll tax basis; contributions to health insurance would be made through work (regardless of the specific employer) into a standardized benefit pool.

A final key value we have to agree on is to recognize and respect Americans' love of technology. Canadians and others like to say that the United States has an extravagant health system that uses technology to revive the nearly dead, with little or no difference in health outcomes. That is being grossly unfair to the American ideals of the frontier and of technological progress. Americans really do like the machines that go ping. Americans value technological intervention to solve problems. They respect and value medical progress, and it is unlikely we will ever have a U.S. system in which government fiat prevents cutting-edge technologies from having at least a chance to prove themselves. This contrasts sharply with other cultures, which are much more wary about new technology and are much more accepting of government controls on the systematic diffusion of that technology. Technology assessment, for example, is a much more central part of policymaking in such countries as Sweden and Canada than it is in the United States.

Step Two: Communicate Across Constituencies

There is an astonishing lack of dialogue across the U.S. health care system. Hospitals and health systems are in passive-aggressive engagement with physicians, on the one hand, and managed care plans, on the other. There is little or no effective integration across the system. There are many contracts and relationships but little or no dialogue and meaningful discussion about how to solve each other's problems.

Dialogue across constituencies in health care is similarly constrained and ineffectual. Even within the public health community there is a lack of dialogue among the various players; indeed, there is more competition over who is more righteous than the other than there is sensible dialogue and discourse among the various constituencies.

We need to broaden and strengthen hospital and health system boards and managed care system boards. Hospital boards in particular suffer from the notorious Bronze Plaque Syndrome: raising money for buildings and machines that can benefit from having a bronze plaque attached to them saying "proudly provided by your board of trustees." This behavior reinforces the hospital-centric, technocentric nature of health care and really undermines efforts to focus on the determinants of health. Hospital and health system boards also are not well equipped to deal with economic turmoil. Hospital board members traditionally have signed on to provide and encourage hospitals to develop new technological facilities to make the next generation of CAT scanner or PET scanner or DOG scanner available to the local community. They do not sign on to preside over the mother of all reengineering projects. Consequently, they have a great deal of difficulty making tough choices in the face of economic turmoil. As Bob Leitman, CEO of

Louis Harris and Associates, is wont to say, "It is tough to close the wing of a hospital with your mother's name on it."

We need to focus on building whole and healthy communities. Our local health care leaders need greater focus on strengthening the continuum of care in each community. But, in addition, they must reach out to other partners who play a role in the determinants of the community's health. We need to bring together the constituencies that represent the various elements of the continuum of care (hospitals, physician services, long-term care, and community health resources) and the constituencies who represent the infrastructure for the determinants of health (including churches, schools, local community organizations, employers, and law enforcement organizations).

We can develop an American compromise around healthier communities that is less socialistic than that first originated outside the United States. An American compromise would be more accepting of a role for hospitals both as catalysts in local communities and as providers of health care services. Again it must be stressed that there is a community demand for sophisticated medical services—population health measures won't remove an inflamed appendix or fix a broken leg—and high-quality medical care is one of the key dimensions that community leaders point to as a source of value and benefit for local communities. Hospitals must engage in greater dialogue with these community organizations and find a way for these organizations to participate without the organizations' being subservient to the hospital, on the one hand, or becoming a bunch of whiny diversionaries from the central mission of the hospital, on the other. This is a profound challenge and requires new forums and new vehicles for dialogue across the continuum of care and across the community.

Next, we must create forums for public-private conservation. The public and private sectors in America do not talk to one another nearly as much as they should. In other countries, leaders in both the public and private sectors are peers in an economic sense and in an intellectual sense. There is a tendency in the United States to presume that public sector decision makers are somehow inferior to private sector decision makers. The public sector may be compensated less highly in the United States than it is in other countries, but certainly my experience has been that neurons are more equally distributed between the public and private sectors than the American public believes.

Public-private exchange is essential to resolve many of the challenges facing the health care system and facing health in general. For example, public health officials and managed care should spend more time at the table as the managed care market consolidates and as health plan concerns become synonymous with public health concerns.

Technology companies should be in dialogue with payers, not just with providers. The companies who make technology, be it information technology or pharmaceuticals and medical products, need to have a seat at the table in local communities and need to be involved in dialogue with the various constituencies in health care delivery. However, the trend of the moment is quite the reverse. For example, pharmaceutical companies are less thoroughly engaged with their managed care and health system customers than they have been in the past. Rather, the pharmaceutical companies are now investing in marketing directly to physician influencers and to consumers. Although this may be seen as a healthy thing, it really makes it easier for antagonistic, short-sighted pricing policies to be enacted between pharmaceutical companies and the managed care payers.

Step 3: Focus on Physicians

The U.S. health care system will never be reformed without the active support, participation, and leadership of the country's doctors. Like it or not, physicians are the central caregivers and decision makers in the health care delivery system. U.S. physicians, the most highly trained and compensated on the planet, have made significant improvements in the quality of medical care over the last one hundred years in the United States and around the world. Unfortunately, in the last decade, they have slipped further and further back from their role of leadership into one of passive-aggressive sniping at the health care system for how it fails them. This behavior is not helpful.

Physicians need to be brought back into the mainstream of decision making, but they in turn have to step up to the plate and acknowledge that they have responsibilities in developing a vision for the future for U.S. health care. They are angry and upset. They are trapped like hamsters on the treadmill of discounted fee for service. They are unable to affect the basics of their daily economic existence, whether in terms of prices or quantities. Physicians cannot do anything else for a living that approximates the earnings they can currently make out of medical care, and they're ill equipped for other kinds of roles outside of health care. They are among the most immobile forms of human capital, occupationally and geographically. I once postulated that there was a Reverse Oregon Trail—specialists in covered wagons heading East in search of fee for service. The trail never really materialized simply because there was no wagon train, nobody to lead specialists back to Tennessee or to Erie, Pennsylvania, and, once they got there, nobody really willing to welcome them with open arms. The last thing you need if you're a specialist in the Midwest is some high-income-demanding California specialist coming to town to open up a new practice.

We are looking to U.S. doctors to describe a new vision for the future. No matter what the vision, we need physicians to focus on developing medical managers and medical leaders. Investments made by foundations and others in new programs to improve the quality and capacities of medical leaders are to be applauded, but they are insufficient to deal with the complexity of a medical care industry spending in excess of a trillion dollars annually. There are few places for physicians to get the managerial skills they need to enable them to take their rightful place in organizing and managing what is becoming the largest enterprise on the planet. (Remember that if U.S. health care were a separate economy, it would be the fourth largest in the world.)

Physicians need to experiment with new organizational forms and new forms of reimbursement. There is no clear vision in the medical community of the appropriate form of medical practice nor of the appropriate form of medical reimbursement for the future. There is a hankering for a return to the old days of fee for service, but the vision of the future cannot be a return to the 1960s or the 1970s, and, quite honestly, this imagined golden age was just that: imagined. Physicians' incomes in real terms are at least 20 percent higher today than they were twenty years ago, so physicians are wrong to assume they have economically faltered over the last twenty years. In contrast, real incomes of physicians in many countries, including France, Australia, the United Kingdom, and Canada, have declined over the same period.

What is actually happening is that physicians' incomes and clinical autonomy do not match their expectations and the expectations of continuous improvement that they inherited from their forebears. Physicians need to experiment with new organizational forms just like every other form of enterprise has had to do, professional or not. There are models and metaphors everywhere for physicians to examine:

- Large consulting companies in which partners routinely have incomes in excess of a million dollars annually
- Law practices that increasingly use paralegal and other auxiliary professionals
- Advertising and other professional services firms that have a much looser and more freewheeling style of decision making
- Team-based architecture and design organizations in which the formal training of individuals is less important than the combined organizational expertise brought to bear to deliver a particular service

These organizational forms all provide seeds of experiments for twenty-first-century practice. Where are the experiments in the physician community? Medical practice is astonishingly conservative and, in an era of rapid change in other businesses, seems incredibly resistant to innovation.

Most important then is that physicians need to provide a vision of change and to be personally willing and able to make these changes. There are some very interesting opportunities, particularly with the feminization of medicine and the increasing role women are going to play in medicine in the future. We need to see stronger and stronger linkages between physicians and other health professionals, who also are mostly women. Team building and community building are likely to occur more effectively under the helm of female physicians than under that of male physicians.

Step 4: Engage Consumers Honestly

We have to tell the truth about technology and disease, about what works and what doesn't work, about what really contributes to health and what doesn't, and about the role that various health behaviors, health actions, and organizational and economic policies have on the health status of individuals and communities. Right now no one is telling those truths. Indeed, a whole host of actors—medical professionals, pharmaceutical companies, those in the left proposing socialized reforms, and those offering alternative medicine, among others—are systematically providing disinformation. Not everyone is receiving a fair hearing, nor are there really truth and honesty about the particular relative merits. Here there is an enormously important role for private foundations and other agencies that can fund careful scholarship to tease out the truth about technology, disease, health status, and health behavior. But before these research investments are made, it is important that we talk about the consequences of the results. If we find that certain technologies or certain proposed interventions—be they technological or policy interventions, be they politically correct or not—don't work or have limited value, then we must make policy that reflects that truth. We should not simply cave in to new, supposedly better ideas that are founded on ideology or professional bias—medical savings accounts (MSAs) being a classic example.

We should have public debate about conflicting health care values, a debate that incorporates the variety and diversity of opinion across this country. Many Americans believe passionately that health care is a right. Many share the opposing view that it is a privilege. We need to recognize that there is no mainstream consensus around these issues. We need to help consumers in honestly debating differences in their values. For example, in recognizing that tiering is something that many people accept and are particularly comfortable with in health care and in other social services, we need to further focus people on helping design specific floors and ceilings in health care that are acceptable. How much tiering is tolerable? We need to have an honest consumer debate about what is an acceptable level of service as a basic floor and how much variation and difference between rich and poor we are going to tolerate.

The Oregon Medicaid Plan confronted the beast of rationing. Oregon was an interesting experiment in which policymakers (with community input) rank-ordered medical procedures on the basis of cost-effectiveness. Items on the bottom of the list were simply not covered so that highly cost-effective preventive measures would be covered. Rationing is certainly one of the major issues about which we have to engage consumers honestly. More broadly, though, the rationing debate is really about both the potential and the limits of new technology and about how that technology affects the health care delivery system, particularly in caring for the very old and terminally ill. These are incredibly difficult questions that require a much more honest debate than we have engaged in so far.

Oregon also taught us that it is important to frame questions about designing the floor. If we accept that everyone has a right to a basic plan, how basic is basic? That, again, is one of the brave notions behind the Oregon model. In Oregon, policymakers tried to do it on the basis of identifying clinical interventions that "made the cut" in terms of cost-effectiveness. This approach is troublesome because the history of health services research indicates that clinical interventions are not necessarily cost-effective per se; rather, their cost-effectiveness depends very much on the clinical context in which they are applied. For example, one must ask, What is the prevalence of disease within the particular group? What are the clinical indications? What are the likely outcomes with or without intervention? Cimetidine is a very useful therapy for people with ulcers. It is a less cost-effective therapy if it's used for people with upset stomachs, and indeed part of the overall success of Cimetidine and Tagamet (its brand-name form) was that it became Rolaids for yuppies, not because it was used exclusively to treat stomach ulcers.

Step 5: The Vision Thing

We must develop the capacity to think ahead and develop new ideas. We are quite clearly in a crisis of theory right now. There is an absence of vision. Where to go next? We need to reenergize visionary leadership. We need to return to a spirit of experimentation in U.S. health care. We need a new leadership agenda. We need leadership training, cross-sector internships that allow people from various sectors both inside and outside health care to participate in varied settings and gain a broader perspective on health care.

We need to take advantage of the growth of the Internet and the merging possibilities for e-commerce in health care. We must encourage local communities to create solutions for themselves. Although universality cannot be solved locally, huge improvements can be made by local community stakeholders working together.

We need to engender long-term thinking among our leaders and among all who work in health care organizations, and we need to recognize that good governance creates good leadership. We therefore must develop boards and organizational structures that encourage long-term thinking.

The health care industry needs to innovate. We need to encourage new experiments in policy and in the marketplace. Ideally, in the new millennium we will have a wave of reform that leads to a new U.S. health care system—a system that is compassionate, innovative, effective, and sustainable. We can do better. We will do better.

Afterword

Health care and the world have changed profoundly in the last two years since this book was written. Yet many of the trends and issues identified in the text remain in force. Some have become amplified, like the call for defined-contribution health plans in the wake of rapidly rising corporate health care costs. Some have diminished, such as physician practice management companies and the growth in the Medicare+Choice program. New trends have come to the fore such as concerns over the nursing shortage, and prescription drug pricing and marketing. Other trends have come and gone in the space of two years: the Internet and e-health chief among them. I hate to say I told you so.

I stand by the text you have read. While there may be some errors in fact or judgment, I have not changed my point of view about almost all of what was written two years ago. As I say to my clients, one of the benefits of being a futurist is you never have to change your slides.

Still, much has changed in health care. And, of course, the entire world changed on September 11th. This Afterword is an attempt to look again at the future of health care through the lens of emerging reality, to update some of the long term trends, and to examine what September 11th means for the long-term future of health care. As before, I try to analyze those trends but more importantly draw conclusions for organizational strategy and individual leadership.

September 11th and the Beginning of the New Future

I first came to New York in 1964. I was eleven and a half (back when halfs mattered). I came with my family from Scotland on a cruise to New York's World Fair. (Lest this leads you to illusions of

my grandeur, I should explain that my father was a young archi-
tect, and it was a cheap cruise. I believe we were on F deck and the
boiler room was on C deck.)

I will never forget, as long as I live, sailing into the New York
harbor on a magnificent summer morning. I have had a love affair
with New York City ever since. I have many friends and business
associates in New York, and I spend a lot of time there. Indeed, I
was scheduled to fly to New York from San Francisco on September 11th until my meeting got cancelled (fortunately) a day or two
before the tragedy. Like all of us who love New York and New Yorkers, I was horrified by the events and moved by New Yorkers' hero-
ism in response. We will never forget that day.

I returned to New York exactly one month later, on October
11th, visiting Ground Zero with my longtime New York friend
and business partner, Bob Leitman. Even when you see the dev-
astation with your own eyes it is hard to believe that it happened
and that anyone could perpetrate such horror on people simply
going to work.

September 11th has changed everything in world affairs and
the economy. It has shaped public opinion about patriotism,
presidents, and politicians, and it has transformed national and
personal priorities. America is now engaged in a long-term battle
against terrorists, who feed off the globally disaffected and spit
their venom at the West. American foreign policy and national
budget priorities are obviously changed for the foreseeable future.

The economy will be rocky for some time as uncertainties pre-
vail for government, business, and households. But America and
the world will recover stronger and more united in the long run.

The major impact of September 11th for the health care industry is the new budget reality faced by the Bush administration.
There was no budget surplus before September 11th, and because
the global economy was dealt a major blow by Bin Laden, there is
no budget surplus after September 11th. At the same time, there
have been huge new public expenditures required to make airlines
secure, postal systems safe, and our public health systems strong
enough to weather the threats of bioterrorism. All this is in addition to the required public investment in military, diplomatic, and
homeland security priorities. This new budget reality crowds out
health care both financially and politically for some time to come.

America's unity and bipartisanship in the face of terrorism could spill over into the domestic arena and usher in a new era of moderation, cooperation, and progress. Alternatively, politicians like to fight, and while it is patriotic to unite on national security issues, domestic policy matters may become the venue for bitter partisanship. What actually plays out remains to be seen, but I am not betting on the "Kumbaya" scenario.

The events of September 11th have other, longer term effects on health care. For example, terrorism has fueled the social insecurity of an aging baby boom. We boomers lost all of our 401K money in the bubble of 2000, and with layoffs and bioterrorism threats, the average worker is feeling less secure. This may lead to the creation of new employee benefits (paid for by the individual but organized by the employer, so-called voluntary benefits). The prevailing sense of insecurity will likely make health benefits an even more important issue for unions.

Perhaps the most lasting effect of the war on terrorism is the recognition that big government is important. The safety of our air transportation and postal systems, and our public health system as first line of defense against bioterrorism, are big government functions. The public health system has languished over the last few years, particularly at the county and state level, because other direct service issues of serving the uninsured have swamped state and local government agencies. The revitalization of public health has now become a national priority.

Although everything changed on September 11th, all of the driving forces shaping health care that existed before are still evident, and it is these driving forces and their effects that are the focus of this Afterword.

An Update on Values

George Bush was elected with a majority in the Electoral College and the Supreme Court, but not in the popular vote. The closeness of the election mirrors the almost equal division in the country. Half of Americans are conservative and the other half are Canadian. It is this lack of consensus on ideological issues such as universality and equity in health care that makes it difficult to envisage a single-payer government solution any time in the future. The mechanics of policy in Canada, France, or Germany, and their success in delivering cost-effective health care are irrelevant. Americans are not Canadian. They may be united against terrorism, but they are not united on national health policy.

Nowhere is the tension more evident than in prescription drug coverage for the elderly. We should have coverage for the elderly, and it should be inexpensive, but we don't want to kill innovation and research and development from a vibrant and profitable pharmaceutical industry. To add further layers of irony, most Americans (including many seniors) are also investors in the drug industry, one of the few financial safe havens even in turbulent times. We want the best medicine for everyone but we don't want government to provide it all, and we don't want to limit an individual's freedom to trade up with their own money, and we don't want to eviscerate the drug companies.

A related policy area that illustrates the value tension is the future of Medicare. Politicians of both stripes are reluctant to do much more than pledge their support for maintaining Medicare. But the central question is, What will the program look like in twenty years when the demographics turn nasty? Republicans have advocated for broadening and extending market-based mechanisms such as the Medicare+Choice model. Unfortunately, the market isn't cooperating. Medicare+Choice is in hasty retreat. All the major HMOs that offered Medicare products have trimmed their offerings geographically and increased cost sharing with consumers, particularly for prescription drug coverage. Pundits argue that Medicare+Choice may only survive in three markets: New York, Florida, and California, where there are established players on both the health plan side and the delivery side. In California, Kaiser could have all the Medicare it wants and runs the risk of being selected against by sick seniors seeking low out-of-pocket costs. Mitigating this is the fact that the majority of Kaiser Medicare enrollees are lifetime Kaiser members who age into the program after retirement. Medicare+Choice illustrates the tension in values between those who believe in universal single-payer models and those who believe in competition. The differences are ideological and significant, and will not be resolved easily. The Republicans will be in a difficult ideological spot if the last health plan left standing in the competitive market for Medicare patients is nonprofit Kaiser: this would be the mother of all ironies.

The future of Medicare is part of the broader question of how we as a society will resolve the inevitable tensions between demanding consumers, an aging population and workforce, and incredible new technology? It is too simple to say just pay more for health care: we need to completely redesign it.

The Role of Aging and Technology: 2022 as Target Date

The future of health care is always clear to futurists: it will be different because of aging and technology. We futurists have been saying this for a long time. Yet if you look at American health care from thirty thousand feet what do you see? The over-sixty-five population today accounts for only 13 percent of the total population, up from 11 percent in 1980. We still have a health care delivery system in which physicians see patients for fifteen to twenty minutes and decide what to do based on what the doctor learned in medical school or picked up through continuing medical education. We still have hospitals and nursing homes and physicians offices organized in much the same way they were fifty years ago. True, there are lots of new technologies that allow hospital stays to be shorter and to turn patients' living rooms into intensive care units, but the institutions really haven't changed much. Despite managed care, third parties still pay for health care on a fee-for-service basis. The American health care system has a remarkable ability to resist change. We need to innovate.

And there are powerful forces that will require us to innovate. First, there are the futurist's friends—aging and technology. By 2022 a full 20 percent of the population will be over sixty-five. And they will not be the passive stoics of Tom Brokaw's "Greatest Generation"—they will be cranky, selfish, self-indulgent baby boomers like me. They will want everything and will sacrifice nothing. Armed with information and attitude, they will demand the best that technology can offer. And technology will oblige. The combination of progress in medical science and information technology holds the promise of fabulous new interventions that will be incredibly effective and expensive. We will want it all. Moreover, the fledgling science of genomics will mature to a point where care will have to be customized to my particular gene profile to be most effective.

Will the combination of new science and aging, demanding consumers simply be bolted on to the current chassis of health care financing and delivery? Most health care experts believe this does not compute. We desperately need to innovate.

Innovation is required at the policy level. Who should pay for health care and how? It is fashionable to talk about defined-contribution health plans and consumer-directed health care, but how much tiering in health care will we tolerate as a society? If genomics and genetic testing advance as experts predict, and we will have many tests that accurately predict an individual's likelihood of disease, what does that mean for the concept of experience-related health insurance?

Innovation is required in financing health care. Consumers are going to be more responsible for paying for care but through what mechanisms? Managed care needs to reinvent itself or move aside.

But the greatest innovation must come in the delivery of medical care. Health care needs to redesigned to fully take advantage of advances in information technology, such as the Internet. The medicine of the future needs to be high tech and high touch: it needs to combine the potential efficiency of e-commerce with compassion and caring from motivated professionals.

Such innovation will require real leadership from policymakers, entrepreneurs, and physicians alike. The stakes are high. If we don't innovate it could get ugly.

The New Vision and the Reluctant Donkey

Health care financing and delivery needs to be redesigned over the next twenty years. Why twenty years? As we have seen above, in 2022 the peak of the baby boom turns sixty-five. Fully 20 percent of the population will be over sixty-five, compared with 13 percent today. We will have an aging white population expecting its Medicare to be paid for and delivered by an increasingly uninsured and increasingly minority working population. We will have incredible new technologies and spineless politicians who will promise these technologies to the people without explaining who will pay for them. This does not compute. We can't keep doing what we are doing.

The Institute of Medicine's most recent report, *Crossing the Quality Chasm,* began the twenty-year redesign process with some lofty ideals and practical first steps to cross the quality chasm. It is the best hope we have for a new vision of health care in the new millennium. But the health care system is like a reluctant donkey, stubbornly resisting change. In health care we like to go to meetings about change: we don't like to change. The resistance to change is understandable. The U.S. health care system is bigger than the entire Italian economy. You would not expect the redesign of Italy to be trivial.

The movers and shakers behind the Institute of Medicine (IOM) reports are a policy elite frustrated by the lack of "systemness" in American health care. By first focusing on the patient safety issue, the IOM committee rang the alarm bell on the dysfunction in health care delivery. In *Crossing the Quality Chasm,* the IOM took a step toward articulating the elements of a redesigned future.

The book outlines six basic aims: that care be 1) safe, 2) effective and evidence-based, 3) patient-centered, 4) timely, 5) efficient, and 6) equitable. Simple and sensible as these aims may seem, some are actually quite controversial. For example, evidence-based medicine is still anathema to a lot of AMA surgeon types who ridicule it as cookbook medicine. Similarly, as I have argued throughout this book, Americans are culturally conflicted on the issue of equity. Nevertheless, the IOM did exactly the right thing by laying out the values and principles behind their redesign recommendations.

The IOM book has much to say about how care fails today and how it can be improved in the future. The core of the redesign ethos is embodied in a set of rules for redesign quoted here (Institute of Medicine, *Crossing the Quality Chasm,* p.8):

- *Care based on continuous healing relationships.* Patients should receive care whenever they need it and in many forms, not just face-to-face visits. This rule implies that the health care system should be responsive at all times (twenty-four hours a day, every day) and that access to care should be provided over the Internet, by telephone, and by other means in addition to face-to-face visits.
- *Customization based on patient needs and values.* The system of care should be designed to meet the most common types of needs, but have the capability to respond to individual choices and preferences.

- *The patient as the source of control.* Patients should be given the necessary information and opportunity to exercise the degree of control they choose over health care decisions that affect them. The health system should be able to accommodate differences in patient preferences and encourage shared decision-making.
- *Shared knowledge and the free flow of information.* Patients should have unfettered access to their own medical information and to clinical knowledge. Clinicians and patients should communicate effectively and share information.
- *Evidence-based decision-making.* Patients should receive care based on the available scientific knowledge. Care should not vary illogically from clinician to clinician or from place to place.
- *Safety as a system property.* Patients should be safe from injury caused by the care system. Reducing risk and ensuring safety require greater attention to systems that help prevent and mitigate errors.
- *The need for transparency.* The health care system should make information available to patients and their families that allows them to make informed decisions when selecting a health plan, hospital, or clinical practice, or choosing among alternative treatments. This should include information describing the system's performance on safety, evidence-based practice, and patient satisfaction.
- *Anticipation of needs.* The health system should anticipate patient needs, rather than simply reacting to events.
- *Continuous decrease in waste.* The health system should not waste resources or patient time.
- *Cooperation among clinicians.* Clinicians and institutions should actively collaborate and communicate to ensure an appropriate exchange of information and coordination of care.

In a nutshell, the IOM is looking for a health care system where Charles Schwab meets Nordstroms meets the Mayo Clinic. This report and the efforts it has spurred are our best hope for a better future for health care. But the principles of redesign will not be implemented easily.

We need to flesh out these and other alternate visions of a redesigned future. But more important, we need the leaders who can take us there. We need to celebrate the pioneers who drag the donkey across the chasm, who take the heat in the short run to show us the light in the long run. We have only twenty years, and it is a very big and very stubborn donkey.

An Update on the Driving Forces for Change

While it is impossible to predict the future, it is possible to analyze the driving forces creating change. In health care, several key driving forces remain in place: health industry demonization (managed care and pharmaceuticals in particular), rising consumerism, changing demographics of patient and worker, e-health, and what I am calling the New Principles of Purchasing Health Care.

The Demonization of the Managed Care and Pharmaceutical Industries

The managed care industry continued to be demonized through the election debates of 2000 at all political levels. Every politician had to have a position on the Patients' Bill of Rights. The genius of the Bush campaign was that it took away from the Gore campaign what should have been traditional Democratic issues of protecting Medicare, prescription drugs for seniors, and the Patients' Bill of Rights by convincing the public that Bush, too, had a solution. Surveys at the time showed that the public couldn't tell the positions apart, a fact that may have cost Gore the election.

But the demonization of managed care has gone so far that journalists are almost piling on at this stage. HMOs are only one point away from tobacco companies as the most hated in America, which leads me to the conclusion that CIGNA should just merge with Philip Morris.

The only good news for the managed care companies is that the sights of the media are now firmly trained on the pharmaceutical industry as the new demons in health care. Negative media coverage of the industry's pricing and marketing practices has increased exponentially from 1999 to 2002.

Do not underestimate the effect of industry demonization on both the managed care and pharmaceutical industries. In the case of managed care, the demonization led not only to the Patients' Bill of Rights legislation, but to the strategic reversal of most health

254 HEALTH CARE IN THE NEW MILLENNIUM

plans from tightly managed, closed-panel networks. Instead, every health plan went to open-access products and loosened the controls on hospitals and physicians. Indeed, in surveys conducted in 2001, health plans report that both hospitals and physicians had the upper hand in negotiations over fees. This is a sharp turnaround from the mid-1990s when health plans were ascendant. It is no surprise, then, that costs are headed up again. It also explains why across the country we hear reports of a shortage of specialists. Not only have we demonized managed care but we have demonized the gatekeeper model with it. The return to open networks means a return to specialists over primary care physicians, and perhaps even to a specialist shortage as the medical labor market gets whipsawed by the health care market's changing preferences for care delivery models.

Similar effects of demonization can be seen in the pharmaceutical industry. While still riding high financially, the pharmaceutical industry is very concerned about its image. Industry-wide and company-specific initiatives are under way to improve both the behavior and the image of the industry. For example, Pfizer and Bristol-Myers Squibb both negotiated a "put your money where your mouth is" reimbursement system with the Florida Medicaid program. In exchange for inclusion on the state formulary and in lieu of deep discounts, the companies agreed to provide disease management services that will save hospital and other costs. Similarly, Glaxo Smith Kline and Pfizer are amongst the first companies to offer a voluntary discount card program for seniors. Many more such image-enhancing initiatives will take place in the months and years ahead.

Demonization inevitably leads to changes in public policy and private strategy. The Patients' Bill of Rights would never have been raised had it not been for HMOs becoming the whipping boys of the press. Similarly, the drug industry will have to resolve the Medicare coverage issue or face continued demonization for their pricing and marketing practices.

Evidence-based Consumerism

In most markets, and most industries, organizations are accountable to their customers. If you make a product that doesn't work or doesn't meet customer needs in some other way, then you won't make money, and your shareholders will be unhappy. The magic of market forces makes firms accountable. But markets fail in health care. (By the way, that's why we have a whole branch of economics called health economics, and we don't have dog food economics or Sport Utility Vehicle economics). The major source of market failure in health care, according to the Nobel laureates, is asymmetry of information—in a nutshell, doctors know more than patients. Therefore we have created all kinds of societal institutions like professions, universities, government regulators, health plans, and review organizations in an attempt to make doctors and their workshops more accountable.

With the rise of the Internet and the new sophisticated consumer, some are challenging the asymmetry of information argument and asking why can't health care be like other markets and be accountable to the consumer. These critics have a point. More than a hundred million Americans have surfed the net for health care information, according to pollsters at Harris Interactive. At the same time, consumers are declaring their preferences for complementary and alternative therapy and paying good money for it, out of their own pocket. Isn't that the ultimate accountability?

Before we all get too carried away, let me suggest that there are two types of consumerism, the first of which I would call *naïve market consumerism* (this is Milton Friedman on steroids). Many in the pharmaceutical, medical products, and emerging health insurance markets subscribe to the notion that whatever the consumer wants to spend his or her money on in health care is fine (and by definition utility maximizing for the consumer). So it's the consumer's choice if she decides to lower her cholesterol by getting Lipitor prescribed by her doctor or by purchasing herbal remedies called "The Fat Trapper" and "Exercise in a Bottle" after seeing the infomercial. (Please note, I am not making this up—stay up late enough watching cable TV and you will know of "The Fat Trapper.")

A second form of consumerism is what I would term *evidence-based consumerism*. This makes the consumer a partner in the process of accountability by providing them with the scientifically based support to make informed judgment. It addresses the asymmetry of information head-on and tries to level the playing field.

The explosion in health-related Web sites and self-help resources is assisting consumers in overcoming their anxiety about not knowing enough. But to date, we have not made these information purveyors accountable for their counsel. We lack a system of accountability for health care information.

There are some signs of improvement. The FDA regulates drug information, and so pharmaceutical companies are a reliable source of information about their products, although skeptics may be leery of their aggressive advertising and promotion. Similarly, the professional medical societies are playing a more formal role on the Internet and will bring their professional standards (and biases) to the information exchange. This is not enough. Consumerism needs to be evidence-based, where there is a seal of approval placed on the information, backed up by the same accountability that exists in the peer-reviewed scientific literature. Consumers are showing an appetite for industrial-strength medical Web sites (the kind that real doctors use) that are evidence-based. New organizations such as Medrock (a medical concierge service aimed at helping patients with serious medical conditions), BMJ Unified (a new joint venture between United HealthCare and the *British Medical Journal*), Medem and Medscape (both Web-based businesses with impeccable scientific credentials) may all evolve as pioneers in evidence-based consumerism.

While this is all encouraging, we have a long way to go. Consumers are much more swayed by pharmaceutical direct-to-consumer (DTC) advertisements on TV and in print than they are by report cards on providers and health plans. Indeed in Harris Interactive surveys taken in 2001, a full 30 percent of adults say they have visited their doctors and asked for a specific drug they had seen advertised, some 14 percent had the prescription filled, a phenomenal rate of adoption. In contrast, fewer Americans have seen a comparative report card on either health plans (18 percent), hospitals (22 percent), or doctors (13 percent), and less than 2 percent of Americans have acted on any of that information. We are becoming more evidence-based consumers but we also are subject to the forces of marketing and advertising that we see in other consumer industries.

A key question in this new consumerist world is whether the consumer is actually going to be asked to pay directly out of pocket, either for premiums, deductibles, copayments, and co-insurance charges, reversing a thirty-year trend. The resounding answer seems to be yes, despite employers' reluctance to pursue these strategies in the tight labor market of 1999–2000. As health care premiums escalate in the 10 to 15 percent range for the foreseeable future, employers will be increasingly focused on passing costs on to their employees. Insurance experts say this will be particularly acute in the open enrollment cycle of January 2003, because for many large employers the planning and communications cycle for such major benefit changes begins in the spring of 2002. We will explore the nature of this shift in costs to consumer below in the section on the new principles of purchasing health care.

Changing Demographics of Patient and Employee

Although the American population is aging, we have pointed out throughout this book that the peak of the baby boom, those born in 1957, do not turn sixty-five until 2022. That is why I insist we have twenty years to fix the system. But it is true that all of us boomers are moving into the early stages of total body breakdown: we have been the Advil generation, and we are fast becoming the Claritin, Celebrex, and Lipitor generation as we manage the chronic diseases that emerge in middle age. We also have aging parents who are the heavy users of health care, so, like it or not, the baby boom generation is in the health care consumption business as patients or family members.

But the big surprise demographically has not been the aging effect on the demand for health care, as relentless and predictable as it may be. No, the surprise is the effect on the supply of health care. As the baby bust (those born between 1968 and 1988) moves through, we do not have the same number of young people entering the labor market. This fueled the "war for talent" seen in the economy in the boom days of the millennium. It also explains why unemployment remains around 5 percent, despite a plummeting economy. The worker shortage underpins employers' broader resistance to cutting health benefits until recently. But the most direct and dramatic effect of the worker shortages has hit hospitals in the form of the nursing shortage.

Half of nurses are over fifty, and the age of nursing faculty approaches fifty-seven. Young women interested in clinical careers are pursuing medicine in increasing proportions. Across the country at leading medical schools the majority of first year students are female (as in law school, incidentally). Nurses trained over the last twenty years have left the field to pursue other careers.

The resolution of the nursing shortage will not be easy. It is a global problem. At the extreme, thousands of nurse recruiters from the U.S., Canada, and the U.K. will be pursuing the last available New Zealand nurse, offering outrageous inducements to move. The health care system is responding to increased supply. But nurses will not be attracted back to the harried life of clinical care without a few inducements:

- *Money.* Nursing salaries will continue to rise, fueling further increases in hospital costs.
- *Meaning at work.* Nurses will demand a sense of professional autonomy to bring back meaning to their work.
- *Respect.* The profession needs to be treated with more respect.
- *Quality working conditions.* Hospitals, homes, doctors' offices, and clinics need to be safe and rewarding places to work. Many nurses fear that care has suffered as a result of decades of clinical downsizing and re-engineering. Throughout it all the intensity of care has risen in both the inpatient and outpatient setting, and many nurses here and abroad report that they are "burned out."

The nursing shortage is the single largest issue facing most hospitals across the country. Hospital costs are increasing rapidly again as the effect of the nursing shortage is coupled with rising utilization and the weakening of managed care controls. These challenges will require even more attention in the decade ahead.

The Rise and Fall and Rise of E-Health

E-health, baby! If Austin Powers was in the health care forecasting business, that would have been his clarion cry as the millennium dawned. The IPOs came fast and furious, anythinghealth.com was hot in the market, and the *Industry Standard*—the dot.com establishment trade magazine (now defunct)—declared breathlessly that "Net entrepreneurs are drooling over the prospect of fixing the nation's health care system." Watch out health care, you are about to be transformed.

Well, from January to September 2000 alone, e-health stocks fell an average of 70 percent (down an average of 90 percent from their all-time highs) according to the leading investment analysts. Dr. Koop is on life support. Healtheon/WebMD is no longer the new, new thing. And disintermediators like Neoforma, who were going to change the rules of purchasing medical supplies, are like whimpering puppies called to heel by the big old boys that run the medical supply game.

What happened? At a meeting in San Francisco in late 2000, a number of observers gave their two cents worth on what happened. Larry Leisure, managing partner of Accenture's dot.com launch centers, and a twenty-year health care industry veteran, pointed to the fact that many dot.com upstarts did not pay enough attention to the core questions: Who is the customer, and what will they pay you for? Leisure also cited the lack of industrial-strength information technology and business systems, and a failure of the upstarts to cement meaningful strategic alliances with key industry players.

At a conference of the Health Financial Management Association Meeting in San Francisco on September 18th, 2000, Chris Hector, a principal with health care venture capital leader Acacia Venture Partners, pointed to four factors for the financial collapse:

1. The strength of the legacy companies
2. Technologies in search of a business model (companies focused more on new-fangled products than on serving customer needs)
3. Cheap capital, which created euphoria in the broader dot.com market and lead to stupid decisions by entrepreneurs and fee-obsessed investment bankers
4. Lack of true innovation in business models

Ed Fotsch, the CEO of Medem, the health care Web-hosting company that is sponsored and owned by the leading medical specialty societies, pointed to the arrogance and naïvete of dot.com opportunists who parachuted into the industry without the vaguest clue of how health care is actually delivered.

They are all right. The new guys (the Second Curve) did not respect the legacy players in the industry (the First Curve). The old players (health plans, doctors, hospitals, PBMs, group purchasing organizations [GPOs], pharmaceutical companies, and medical suppliers) simply didn't trust the arrogant new players and refused to just roll over. For example, health plans formed MedUnite to counter the threat of Healtheon. GPOs like VHA and Premier and supply companies like Abbott, Baxter, and J&J, each formed industry Internet exchanges to challenge the new entrants like Neoforma.

Many of the e-health plays only worked on Powerpoint. Few had any real paying customers, let alone any meaningful scale. Lots of us have gone on-line for health care information to be sure. Indeed, my partners at Harris Interactive and Harvard recently conducted a survey for our clients and found that by 2001, 106 million Americans have been on-line to access health care information—up from 70 million in 1999. There is heavy use of the Internet for health care, but is it a business, and has it changed health care delivery? E-health today is like *Encyclopedia Britannica* in the 1950s: a nice place to look up information. We have become cyberchondriacs driving ourselves to distraction in the middle of the night, but we are not really getting what we want from e-health.

Consumers are more sophisticated. In other dimensions of e-commerce—buying a book, ordering theater tickets, reserving tea at the Ritz in London—you can go on-line and do it. (Trust me, I've done them all.) Consumers expect that from e-commerce. Can you make an appointment with your doctor on-line? Can you renew a prescription, e-mail your doctor, get a wheelchair? Although there are businesses doing all of these, they are not mainstream. And the reason is that the new health economy has yet to connect to the old health economy. The future of e-health is not some cyber-doctor in Newfoundland delivering disembodied medical advice and dispensing pills. No, the consumer wants the services connected to local doctors and hospitals. Consumers want e-health delivered locally, connected to their doctors, hospitals, and health plans. And they are not getting it.

Indeed, the Harris/Harvard surveys show a significant (approximately 20 percent) decline in satisfaction amongst consumers with regard to various dimensions of e-health as Table A.1 shows. (In fairness, this is a declining share of a rising base of consumers that has moved from 70 million to 106 million). Nevertheless, the conclusion is important. E-health has been hyped to the point that consumers (not unreasonably) expect it to deliver meaningful e-commerce services.

**Table A.1. Consumers' Use of E-Health:
Is the Bloom Off the Rose?**

	Percentage of People Helped by the Internet		
Type of Help Received	*1999*	*2001*	*Change*
Understanding of own health problems	73	55	-18
Managing personal health care overall	60	40	-20
Improving communications with doctor	51	31	-20
Complying with treatments recommended by doctor	46	31	-15

Source: Strategic Health Perspectives, Harris Interactive/Harvard University, 2001

This is not to say that e-health is dead and over, quite the contrary. Rather, it is a classic case of what I called in my book, *The Second Curve,* Amara's Law (named after my old boss, Roy Amara, who ran the Institute for the Future for more than twenty years). Amara's law, in a nutshell, is that there is a natural human tendency to overestimate the impact of phenomenon in the short run and underestimate the impact in the long run.

E-health can be the platform for the redesign of American health care delivery. It can be part of the new chassis of health care, as David Lawrence, Kaiser Health Plan CEO, says. But it will require leadership, trust building, and real innovation to bring the old health economy and the new health economy together.

Who will win? Perverse as it may seem, the best positioned of all are the group and staff model HMOs. Both Group Health and Kaiser are months away from very significant roll-outs of e-health capabilities that will allow consumers not only to make appointments and renew prescriptions but to interact with physicians electronically through clinical messaging systems. Similarly, Blue Shield of California (again a stalwart of the non-profit health plan world) has demonstrated capability for mass customization in the interaction with their enrollees through mylifepath.com. (Although in surveys consumers are much less interested in the interaction with health plans compared to interaction with their providers.) Similarly, Web companies such as Medem and Medscape/Medical Logic are run by doctors for doctors, and they show promise in being able to provide practical tools that will allow doctors to communicate more effectively with patients.

The next round of e-health is about to begin. Doctors are starting to e-mail patients in significant numbers (we estimate about 13 percent of all doctors have some e-mail contact with patients today). By 2001, almost half of all doctors had Web sites, a third or more had PDAs, and these numbers were rising rapidly.

We must seize the e-health opportunity, not to make money for dot.comers and venture capitalists, but to change health care delivery. Forever.

The New Principles of Purchasing Health Care

New principles are emerging for the purchasing of health care. Overall they lead to a health system that is more heavily tiered, where there is shallower coverage for rising health care costs, and where the kind of care you receive will depend on an individual consumer's income and willingness to pay. In summary the trends are

- *Consumer responsibility for payment.* No matter what, consumers will be asked to pay more toward their care in premiums, copayments, and co-insurance.
- *Consumer choice.* Consumers will have cost-shifting sold to them in the name of choice. It is a variation of what Marie Antoinette said: "Let them eat choice."
- *Knowledge navigation.* With the complexity of choices, consumers will need increased assistance with navigation through these choices.

- *Mass customization.* Consumers will demand customized care, especially if they are paying for it.
- *Technology tiering.* The kinds of care the patient receives, including the technology and quality of care, will be a function of the consumer's willingness to pay.
- *Pay for performance.* Providers will be reimbursed based on objective measures of performance, including clinical outcomes, patient satisfaction, and other clinical performance measures.
- *E-biz processes.* The administration of the health care system and the trends above will be greatly enabled by e-business processes.

These seven trends are evident in the marketplace. The next three are public policy issues that will emerge if these trends go unchecked and unsupported by public policy. But these are pleas for action more than predictions:

- *Portability.* Many of these trends undermine traditional group insurance principles. As the health care marketplace becomes more atomistic, the consumer will need to have portable benefits regardless of employment changes.
- *Community-based risk adjustment.* Experience-rated group health insurance will go into a death spiral if the seven trends above are implemented in the extreme. Some form of community-based risk adjustment is required to prevent the death of health insurance.
- *Universality.* Inevitably, as these trends play out, the moral bankruptcy and illogic of having forty million people uninsured will be exposed.

Consumer Responsibility for Payment

In pure form, defined-contribution health plans are ones in which employees are given a fixed dollar contribution by employers and asked to choose from a range of insurance options or care systems. While it is fashionable to talk about defined contribution as the next megatrend, it may play out in a more prosaic way with consumers simply paying more out of pocket for health care through copayments, co-insurance, and deductibles. Employers jacking up the cost-sharing with employees is defined contribution by stealth. Either way it will represent the reversal of a thirty-year trend in which there has been progressive economic insulation of the consumer from the cost of care. When consumers have to pay more of their own money they will become even more demanding, more skeptical, and more fearful of being left behind. Surveys show that when consumers have to pay for care directly they don't like it one bit, and this attitude spills over into their perceptions of health care quality and their growing dissatisfaction with the health care system more broadly.

The shift from defined benefit to defined contribution will not necessarily be in pure form, to what consultant Bill Rosenberg of Price Waterhouse Coopers calls the "Cash and the Yellow Pages Model." Under this model, employers give their employees a pile of cash toward their benefits and tell them to go fend for themselves. Such a system is rare, certainly among large employers. But there is an emerging continuum of defined-contribution models from the "Cash and the Yellow Pages Model" extreme to more traditional cost-sharing and co-insurance.

Table A.2. Consumer Responsibility for Payment.

Type	Model	Examples
Pure defined contribution	"Cash and the Yellow Pages"	Rare
Self-directed health plans	Pick-a-priced-provider network	Virus, Health Market
Value purchasing	Value selected by employee with employer's help	Leapfrog Group IHA proposals BHCAG
Trade up	Flex or Cafeteria, three-tiered formulary	FEHBP PBM Formularies Point of Service
Cost-sharing	Increased co-payments, deductibles, co-insurance	Traditional indemnity models, MSAs, and high deductible plans

The new paradigm players, such as Sageo and HealthMarkets, are companies which have developed complex consumer-directed marketplaces in which the consumer selects his or her own provider network at previously negotiated prices. These new companies, with heavy venture capital backing and sophisticated management teams, are attempting to redefine the industry under the rubric "self-directed health plans." Although these innovators have some very interesting ideas and features in their offerings, they are gaining little traction in the marketplace, particularly as a wholesale replacement for large employer groups. Their success is limited partly because the new paradigm is a little more complicated and unproven than the old paradigm of simple cost-sharing and co-insurance, and partly because the existing oligopolistic health plans have begun to offer similar features in their new product design. And remember, the existing players already have customers and cash flow.

Some of the new paradigm players may well find a healthy market among small- and medium-sized employers challenged by enormous rate increases in conventional health plan products. These employers may be forced by economic necessity to offer a medical savings account policy at a very low cost to themselves. Such policies will have high-deductible catastrophic coverage and negotiated provider discounts with a wide network of providers. As a plan member you have insurance, but you will pay a lot out of pocket. For many employers the choice is this high-deductible policy for their employees or nothing.

However you define "defined contribution," one thing is clear: the consumer is going to be asked to pay more. Every health plan CEO I have talked to about this has used the same expression: "the consumer needs to have skin in the game," meaning the consumer needs to have some sense of economic participation in health care, particularly at the point of use.

Even though there is an enormous amount of international health economics literature ridiculing user fees as a means of overall cost containment in health care, it is an inherently American idea that you pay at the point of use. There is no free lunch, after all. I would term it the Ross Perot Effect: you can get Americans to do anything for ten bucks. Ross Perot spent ten dollars a vote in his almost successful presidential bid. For ten dollars you can get people to switch to generics or postpone a questionable doctor visit. It appears to be working. Early survey evidence shows that faced with steeper copayments in a multi-tiered formulary, consumers, particularly those with lower incomes, will trade down to a lower cost alternative twice as often as they trade up to the brand name. Whether this contains overall health care costs is a moot point. What it clearly is doing is raising the hackles of consumer and physician alike. Can the political backlash against consumer payment be far away?

More extreme defined-contribution models will proliferate in the right political and economic context—in crude terms, a Republican administration and a recession. We have both. A recession will accelerate the defined-contribution trend because corporate America has run out of managed care tools. Giants such as GE have been there, done that, bought the t-shirt when it comes to forcing employees into managed care. The next step is empowering consumers: as we said earlier, "you're on your own, pal!"

Corporate America has always provided health benefits reluctantly. It was tax-efficient compensation, but few corporations would claim that managing health benefits is a core competency. Most would like to be rid of the responsibility if they could only trust the government or someone else to do right by their employees. However, the employer-based health insurance system remains immensely popular with the public and with politicians. The politicians are off the hook for payment, and the public (those lucky enough to have insurance) see it as a perk they don't pay for. Employer-based health insurance won't go away easily. It just may be transformed to a heavily cost-shared model over the next few years.

Defined contribution will accelerate according to what my colleagues and I in Strategic Health Perspectives have called the Health Insurance Misery Index. Modeled after Jimmy Carter's stagflation index, it appears as follows:

Health Insurance Misery Index =
Unemployment Rate + Premium Inflation Rate

Our argument is that when the Misery Index approaches 20 percent, health care costs become a CFO- and CEO-level issue for large employers, and major changes in corporate health benefits are made as a result. The last time the index neared 20 percent was in the late 1980s and early 1990s, motivating corporate America to force employees into managed care. Expect defined contribution to grow fast if the numbers exceed 20 percent. Many economists anticipate that the 20 percent barrier could be broken in 2002 or 2003 because premium inflation in the low- to mid-teens is anticipated, and unemployment could exceed 6 to 7 percent in a deep recession.

No matter what, we are going to see a more heavily tiered health care system as a result of the shift to consumer payment. Some employers will resist it because they are heavily unionized or have expensive and scarce knowledge capital embodied in their employees. Others, such as small businesses, service businesses with thin margins, and employers who are struggling financially, will embrace the trend through necessity. Companies such as Polaroid have announced massive shifts to defined contribution as a part of their Chapter 11 bankruptcy reorganization.

And this tiering will have an effect on the care received. An employee's ability to pay out of pocket will shape the service they get, the choices available, the network of providers available to them, and the technology they receive. It may have a direct effect on their health outcomes as a result. It remains to be seen whether the inevitable inequities of tiering lead to a political backlash.

Consumer Choice

Consumer payment and tiering will be sold in the name of choice. But choice of what? Consumers want choice of provider, to be sure. They are uncomfortable with closed-panel arrangements unless they are life-long group practice HMO types. Similarly, consumers prefer a choice of health plan.

Increasingly, consumers will be *forced into* making more complex choices about benefit design that encompass deductibles, copayments, co-insurance, provider networks, formularies, and so forth. The number of choices will be huge. CIGNA HealthCare alone claims to be able to structure and support administratively some four thousand different employee health benefit designs. With all this complexity, communication to employees is going to be an enormous challenge. And with little experience, actuaries, employee benefit managers, and consumers themselves will be finding their own way. It seems inevitable that the coming myriad of choices will turbocharge the sources of market failure in health insurance: moral hazard (when you have insurance you use it); adverse selection (you buy it when you know you are going to need it); and cream skimming (we won't sell it to you if you really need it).

The positive hope is that the combination of choice and consumer payment will lead to more discriminating consumers who will make informed decisions based not just on cost but on value. These consumers will trade off price and costs against value, convenience, outcome, and so forth. Let's keep our fingers crossed. More likely is that consumers will see this as yet another failure of the health care system to meet their needs, and the HMOs may well get the blame again.

Consistent with this trend, several insurers are introducing tiered-network copayments for hospitals. For example, under such arrangements, Hospital A might charge $1,100 for a specific procedure, and Hospital B might charge $2,100 for the same procedure, with no measurable differences in quality. Under these new schemes, the consumer would have to pay a $100 deductible for Hospital A and perhaps a $500 deductible (or half of the difference) for Hospital B. This is plausible when the bill is $1,100. What about when it's $50,000?

There is no question that having "skin in the game" in this very direct way will redefine choice. The question is, will it improve the performance, accountability, and cost-effectiveness of the health care system or will it expose sick people to economic hardship and egregious marketing practices? How will this all work out for the poor, the old, and the chronically ill? The answer inevitably will be *not well.*

Knowledge Navigation

Consumers need help navigating through a myriad of new choices. Scorecards might help but they are not enough. The choices we have to make in health care are just part of the broader choices that we have to make, especially in fields such as energy, education, long distance telephone services, and so forth where choices were once easy and automatic. Tom Philp of the editorial board of the *Sacramento Bee* has pointed to this as choice fatigue: we are exhausted by the time we have picked through the options. The lack of pick up in the choice-laden new paradigm health plans may be a symptom of choice fatigue. Whatever happened to simplicity?

Choice will require better tools for comparison shopping, and health plans, private foundations, and other rating agencies will increasingly provide the data. We must be particularly concerned about assisting the elderly, the poor, and those patients who have different languages and cultural preferences in making these choices.

Perhaps the most important tool of knowledge navigation is the rise of what I have termed the medical concierge. An anecdote will illustrate the general point. A number of primary care physicians with high-rolling patients in my community (Menlo Park/Palo Alto) have abandoned the health insurance system. They are now in the medical concierge business (my term not theirs). They agree to provide basic primary care services to their patients. They are available 24/7 by e-mail, voice-mail, cell phone. They will help the patients and their families navigate through the health system. But, if you require surgery or even some fancy scans you had better have health insurance. They don't want anything to do with insurance and provide the concierge services for a $200 monthly fee billed to your credit card. Variants on this model are springing up all over the country. Before any doctor reading this runs out and starts such a practice, let me point out that there are not enough rich people to go around.

The real lesson of the medical concierge model is that health plans, group practices, or even hospitals need to provide this service embedded in their offerings, for a few dollars a month, using new technology such as the Internet. There are some start-up medical concierge services such as Medrock who are focused on helping very sick patients with complex conditions navigate through the system. Medrock provides a glimpse of service offerings of the future.

Mass Customization

Consumers are more skeptical and demanding in general. When they have to pay with their own money they will get very picky indeed. They will not pay more unless the care works for them and is customized to their needs, values, and preferences. They are going to want care *anywhere, any time, any place*. The diversity of cultures, care preferences, lifestyles, and conditions will require that health care providers and health plans be capable of mass customization.

Genomics is a critical factor behind the coming mass customization of care. Genomics will yield new tests that tell us all about our future course of disease and health. But more important than the burden of prescience (which we futurists carry with us all the time), consumers will know that their care will be more effective if customized for them. *The right drug, for the right patient, at the right time* will become the mantra reinforced by the pharmaceutical industry and the morning shows.

Randy Scott, founder and CEO of Genomic Health , wrote recently about the confluence of three powerful technology forces for change in health care. These are 1) Moore's law (the number of circuits per chip doubles every eighteen months), 2) Metcalfe's Law (the power of the network is proportional to the square of the number of participants), and, 3) what Scott calls The Law of Finite Biology (all biological systems have a finite and thus knowable number of proteins, pathways, and so on). Together these forces will require the health care delivery system to redesign itself from an artisan delivery system of uneven quality to a system of mass customization: efficient, effective, and tailored to the individual needs, preferences, and genetic makeup of individuals.

Genomics will offer new tools of drug discovery, drug development, and customized clinical care. It will change the daily routine of all health care providers. At its extreme, the genomics revolution could lead to a health care system founded on public health, prevention, primary care, and prescription drugs rather than one centered on hospitals and proceduralists.

Technology Tiering

Perhaps the most troubling of all the trends described here is the coming variation in the technical content of care depending on the patient's ability to pay. While it is illegal to treat patients differentially inside the hospital based on their insurance status or ability to pay, we are seeing growing evidence of tiering of technology in the ambulatory environment, in dentistry and cosmetic surgery, and with prescription drugs.

I experienced a stark example of this at a routine visit to my dentist for teeth cleaning. My dental hygienist, a very forceful young Asian lady, told me I had deep pockets. I thought she meant financially, and indirectly she did mean that. She explained that she could place a little antimicrobial chip (about two millimeters square) underneath the gum of the offending tooth, and it would help my deep-pocket problem. Oh, by the way, she said, this little thing costs $43. A pure play add-on. Of course I went for it.

The three-tiered formulary (which is rapidly becoming a five-tiered formulary) is the technology tiering metaphor for the future. The higher the tier the more the consumer has to pay in copayment or (increasingly) in co-insurance terms. Typically the tiers would be structured with copayments such as $5, $10, $15, $25, $50. But even in the top case the copayment may be only 25 percent of the PBM's ingredient costs. In the five-tiered formulary, pioneered originally by the PBM Express Scripts, the tiers are as follows (our labels not theirs):

- Tier 1. Old generics, usually low cost.
- Tier 2. New generics, more expensive, often recently off patent with lots of marketing and advertising support behind them from the drugmakers.
- Tier 3. Rebatable brands. Branded drugs for which the manu- facturers have negotiated a discount with the PBM and/or health plan.
- Tier 4. Non-rebatable brands. Branded drugs for which there is very little rebate or none.
- Tier 5. Lifestyle or discretionary drugs. Drugs such as Claritin or Viagra that are perceived in many cases to be "feel good" rather than medically necessary.

The key to these new formularies is tiers 3, 4, and 5. Tiers 3 and 4 are not necessarily based on relative scientific merit or clinical effi- cacy, but rather on the commercial arrangements made between the pharmaceutical companies and the PBM.

These formulary tiers (tier 5 in particular) mirror the James Brown Effect described earlier: Americans need to pay out of pocket before they can say "I feel good."

Early studies of the effects of this tiering suggest that con- sumers are confused and annoyed by the copayments. Doctors are experiencing a new hassle factor analogous to the early days of utilization review in managed care. Growing numbers of doctors report in surveys that they are prescribing less-than-optimal drugs for their patients. PBMs are accused of gaming the system to increase their rebate income at the expense of their employer clients. This issue will become more rancorous over time and may be the source of more media and, potentially, regulatory attention. But the tiering of drugs is just the beginning. It will spread to hospitals and physician networks in the next generation of health plan design.

Consumers will be asked to trade up with their own money for superior technology. While it's harder to see how the technical content of inpatient care will be easily tiered ("Will that be the $1,000 or the $2,000 stent, Mrs. Johnson?"), the trend is there. It is inherently American: you pay for the upgrade with cash or frequent-flyer miles.

We are moving toward a system of floors and ceilings. We Americans want a floor below which no American falls and the right to trade up with our own money. New economy entrepreneurs, innovative health insurers, and pharmaceutical executives are all salivating at the prospect of serving the affluent clients who can, and will, trade up to these new ceilings. Although our survey-based analysis suggests that the number of trade-up players who are willing and able to trade up is less than 10 percent of the population, amongst the chronically ill—the heavy users of health care—the proportion is even smaller.

Further, the new world of customized, consumerized, and tiered health care will all unravel politically, economically, and morally if we do not guarantee the floor for all Americans. The business of health care must make a case for universality. Without it, the new consumerist nirvana can neither be created nor sustained.

Pay for Performance

Just as the consumer will be asked to pay more for seemingly better care, so providers will be paid more for seemingly better care. These simple market-based principles will go hand in hand. It has long been the goal of managed competition that better performing plans would win economically (by getting a larger market share or higher prices). It never really happened that way because the plans were so undifferentiated, but the idea was nice if you believe in markets. As health plans have become commodities with the same networks of providers, pay for performance is moving to the provider level. This will require much more sophisticated and detailed metrics of provider performance than ever before. There are a number of important pioneering experiments that will get broader application over the next few years. They include

- *The Leapfrog Group.* A group of very large and sophisticated health care purchasers are trying to pay hospitals differentially based on clinical performance measures.
- *The Integrated Health Care Association (IHA) Pay for Performance Initiatives.* The California-based IHA is a public policy group composed of payer, provider, and plan alike. They are pioneering a pay-for-performance system for medical groups in which better-performing medical groups would receive higher capitation payments based on clinical performance, outcomes, and patient satisfaction measures.
- *The Buyers Health Care Action Group (BHCAG) Model.* Minneapolis-based BHCAG is a coalition of employers with 100,000 enrollees in Minneapolis. Enrollees select a medical group (or care system). Each medical group declares itself to be at one of three specific price points quoted in dollars per member per month. The consumer can select from any group, and the provider can position themselves at any of the three price points (most providers and consumers pick the middle band). Consumers are furnished with user-friendly information on the cost, quality, and service offerings of the group. It seems to work well enough, but it is not taking either Minneapolis or the nation by storm.
- *Wellpoint.* California-based Wellpoint has announced it will pay physicians' bonuses based not on containing costs but on improving quality as measured by customer satisfaction. Other insurers have followed.

All of these models are worth watching. More pay-for-performance initiatives will emerge. The intent is to make provider reimbursement a function of performance in medical and service terms, a laudable goal. The implementation requires enormous amounts of information, much of which is impossible to gather and harder still to analyze properly, but we have to start somewhere, and the direction is clear.

But the way in which consumers judge performance is not just a function solely of the scorecards on quality but how the patient feels about the entire customer experience.

I grew up in Britain, in the Basil Fawlty school of customer service—customer as scum—which probably explains my low-level Maslowian view of most service businesses. I don't need to self-actualize at my bank: I just need them to clear the checks I write (yet even this they find challenging).

All services should at least meet the basic Maslowian need of safety. Safe schools, safe airlines, and safe hospitals should be a goal. The brilliance of the patient safety movement was that it set up a discussion about the lack of systems in health care by appealing to the most basic of needs. Great service companies like Charles Schwab or Starbucks have great systems (the information systems and the organizational capacity) to deliver consistent quality.

Beyond safety, most of us look for competence. Is the technical quality there? That's harder to judge in health care: How do we know if our doctor does it right? Despite all the scorecards, most of us judge on subjective factors. Many patients in surveys claim to have changed doctors because they were dissatisfied with quality. It probably was not based on systematic analysis of the technical quality of the care, rather that the physician didn't connect with the patient, didn't spend enough time with them, didn't seem to care.

Comfort and convenience matter. The physical environment of health care is often intimidating, and caregivers are so harried they often don't have time to make the patient feel comfortable. But why do we agonize over the nursing shortage and not over a bank teller shortage? This is because banking has redesigned itself, with ATMs, to serve customers more efficiently. We have not redesigned health care delivery to maximize quality, customer service, and caring.

Caring is the key part of the health care experience. I am not talking about an affable bedside manner. I don't want an excessively cheerful surgeon kneeling by my bedside saying "Hi, I'm Bob. I'll be your surgeon today." God forbid that we turn the bedside into the same insincere, way-too-perky customer service we get in chain steakhouses.

I want caregivers who recognize that I am vulnerable. No matter how smart, well informed, and empowered I may be as patient, friend, or family member, when I come in contact with the health care system I am frightened, anxious, and in pain.

Health care systems need to transform health care delivery to match the best of breed of the service industry in safety, competency, and consistency of customer service. But as we embark on the grand redesign of health care over the next twenty years, let us not neglect the caring part of the health care experience. We need to reduce medical errors, but we also need compassion, connection, and concern.

E-Business Processes

Health care has an immature information technology infrastructure compared to most service businesses. The death of the dot.com phenomenon also sucked much of the venture capital and new ideas out of the e-health bubble. The problem remains, however, as we have seen above: consumers want high-tech high-touch e-commerce from their health care providers. Realizing this, many enlightened health plans are aggressively pursuing what are variously termed B2B, B2C, B2E, and B2B2C opportunities. Health plans and the employers they serve have figured out that if they are to move to a choice-laden environment where the employee/consumer is selecting amongst options, the Internet is the best way to enable these choices through employee self-service applications. Providers, too, are embracing the Internet as a tool for research and patient education.

There are really seven futures for the use of e-commerce in health care.

1. *Limited cyberchondria.* This is the stage we are already at where consumers and doctors use the Internet primarily as a library for information.

2. *AOL for doctors.* This was the WebMD illusion in its original strategy, that somehow doctors would be on-line watching ads from pharmaceutical companies. Doctors don't have enough time to see patients let alone watch ads.

3. *Bloomberg of health.* Similarly, doctors are different from financial executives in that while information is the currency of medicine, doctors don't have the same need for broadcast specialty news that the financial markets have. This model is unworkable also.

4. *Bettyware.* Betty is the most important person in American health care administration. Betty works for the doctor (actually there are four Bettys for every doctor). She keeps the formularies straight, photocopies your insurance card at reception, and spends her day faxing pieces of paper back and forth trying to coordinate care and get paid for it. (It may be terribly politically incorrect to call it Bettyware, but it is factually correct because most back-office workers in physician offices are female, and some, not all, are called Betty). The new WebMD, firmly under the control of Marty Wygod, the entrepreneur who built Merck-Medco, is trying to position itself as the mother of all Bettyware companies. Similarly, MedUnite, a consortium of several health insurers (formed out of fear of the young WebMD), is trying to build much-needed Bettyware solutions for eligibility verification, claims adjudication, and provider credentialing.

5. *Doctors' shopping network.* There was a hope at one time that the new infrastructure of Internet exchanges would eliminate traditional supply-purchasing channels for doctors and hospitals alike. As we discussed above, and like in most industries, the old guard resisted incursions by the e-health start-ups.

6. *E-practice.com.* New applications for physician practice management began to emerge on an Application Service Provider model for medical practice management, medical transcription, and electronic medical records. The euphoria around ASPs was short-lived, and practice management remains the purview of a few established medical software vendors who are trying to put an e-spin on ancient legacy systems. Pharmaceutical companies and their partners (emerging ASPs who provide hand-held PDA prescription ordering solutions to physicians) are a plausible starting point for a wireless, Web-enabled infrastructure, which is where we clearly need to go in the long run.

7. *Platform for e-health redesign.* The hope was that the Internet could be one of the important building blocks of the redesign in health care. That hope remains, but much work needs to be done

to integrate the Internet and computing generally into the redesign of clinical practice.

Often a breakthrough in the use of technology is enabled by industry standards, for example, the explosion of faxes, in the 1980s; Microsoft's hegemony in operating systems and desktop applications in the 1980s and the 1990s; and of course, the HTML, www., dot.com thing. The passage of HIPAA has put the entire health care system on notice that the electronic infrastructure of health care needs an upgrade. HIPAA may provide the much-needed boost to create standardized industry infrastructure, but as I have facetiously suggested to clients overwhelmed by the cost and complexity of complying with the new laws, it may be just easier to ignore HIPAA and do the jail time.

Information technology can be a powerful factor in the redesign of health care delivery over the next twenty years. But a key impediment that HIPAA and the Internet cannot overcome easily is the lack of clinical usage of computers.

There's No Screen

Techno-futurists are full of it. Technology doesn't cause anything. It amplifies, distorts, leverages, and attenuates, but it does not determine the direction of things. It neither creates flattened organizations nor hierarchical ones. It is neither the cause of centralization nor of decentralization. Technology in general (information technology in particular) is neutral in both a geographic and organizational sense.

This was the guts of my Ph.D. dissertation almost twenty years ago. Like most dissertation writers, I was so sick of it when I finished that I didn't want to look at it again, let alone publish it or talk about it with anyone. So I was delighted when a friend passed along to me *The Social Life of Information* by John Seely Brown and Paul Duguid of Xerox PARC fame. The guts of their argument is more wide-ranging, more scholarly, better written, and more readable than my dissertation, but the stance is the same. Futurists and technologists invest too much faith in technological determinism and not enough in the importance of the social context of technological change.

Becoming digital in health care will require much more than computers and bandwidth. It will require the correct social, political,

and economic context and the organizational and personal transformation to bring out the best in the machines. And the transformation needs to make health care truly better not just appease the
technologists.

In just one day, I was reminded of how far we have to go. At 7:00
A.M. I was on the phone with the CEO of a data-mining company
that has successfully applied sophisticated data-mining and pattern-
recognition technology to the oil exploration business. The CEO,
a cancer survivor, wants to "apply the [data-mining] technology to
health care so that doctors could have a synthesis of all the best
information available to them on the screen as they treat the
patient." "What screen?" I asked. "There's no screen. No books
even," I said. "Doctors don't think like that. They like to make it up
as they go along. It's hypothetico-deductive reasoning at best, not
calculus." He was a scientist, and that got him.

Fast forward an hour. I am going for a second opinion about
whether I need neck surgery for a herniated disk. A week ago, the
head of neurosurgery at Stanford University told me I need it, and
I believed him, but hey I'm supposed to be an informed consumer,
so I'm going to the high-priced sports medicine guys who don't do
surgery, and I'm going to be seen by a non-interventionist neurologist. Fancy office buildings, beautiful art, smart staff, yet the same
American health care ritual at reception: they took a photocopy of
my insurance card. (Wouldn't it seem sensible to make the cards
swipeable or something? No Bettyware here.) I get ushered into
an exam room, give the nurse the history, and after a bit of a wait,
the neurologist bounds in. He does a lot of touchy-feely exams, he
asks me questions, he goes into trance-like reflections at times.
He hits me with a little rubber hammer all over the place, including between the eyes. There's no screen.

I came to him hoping to be told that I didn't need surgery.
He told me I did, and immediately. I don't need the screen. I
trust him.

A couple of hours later, after I cancel all my obligations for
the next few weeks, I'm on another conference call. This time it's
with senior officers of the American Heart Association, the NIH,
and the U.S. Public Health Service talking about a conference
they are organizing next year on cardiovascular health. The goal
of the conference is to help a wide range of practitioners and

public health folks discuss ways to reach the healthy 2010 goals set by the Surgeon General. Among the wide range of problems we discussed one was clear: the lack of compliance by patients and physicians with the existing knowledge about cardiovascular health and management of disease. An eminent cardiologist who was participating in the conference call and who is head of a large group practice explained how in his practice the cardio-vascular care guidelines pop up on the screen to remind the doc-tor at discharge about the appropriate follow-up care. The American Heart Association is making these guidelines widely available on the screens of all physicians who want them.

There are screens, and doctors are increasingly using them. But the screens must enhance the science and magic of medi-cine. They must help, not hinder, the connection between physi-cian and patient.

The Three Policy Principles

As we stated earlier, the trends toward new principles of pur-chasing health care are evident in the marketplace but they will unravel unless public policy solutions are found.

Portability

Health policy needs to be adjusted to fit the New Economy in which most people no longer work for large businesses for a lifetime but rather shift employment many times in their career. The vast major-ity of people who change health plans do so involuntarily because of change in employment circumstances: either they changed jobs or the employer changed health plans. We need to build a system of portable benefits, in which workers can move between positions without being exposed to what was once termed job lock. The leg-islation to guarantee issuance of insurance is not enough. Insurance needs to be affordable and portable. Part of the portability prob-lem is that many workers patch together a living with part-time and temporary work while they attend school, pursue their passions, or simply struggle to survive economically. Many of the uninsured are young working people in between parents and permanence. They are not paying for health care nor are they, in the main, using it. But in countries such as Holland or Germany where health insurance is paid for on a payroll tax basis, even temporary and part-time workers contribute to the costs of health care through a payroll tax.

Community-Based Risk Adjustment

The growth in high-deductible health plans, medical savings accounts, and other forms of consumer-pay models will quickly undermine the traditional group health insurance pools. As we discussed in Chapters Seven and Twelve, market-based or policy-based solutions to the problem of risk adjustment need to be found. Absent appropriate risk-adjustment mechanisms, American health care will not be able to develop appropriate reimbursement and incentives for the management of chronic conditions, which is perhaps the central problem of health care for the next twenty years. Without risk-adjustment tools, group insurers may find themselves in a death spiral as healthy risks gravitate to high-deductible plans. Left to its own devices the health insurance market will unravel.

Universality

It seems likely that there will be a backlash against tiering. The consumer-pay trend will fuel inequity in American health care, and the public will notice it. The pay–as-you-go model will raise public fears about being left out of the system and may lead us to a longer term discussion of universal coverage. In the short term this is unlikely. We ought to be talking about it, but we won't until the inequities get so extreme, and the middle class feels so vulnerable, that they react politically. But we do not have another idea in the wings, beyond let the consumer pay more. Again, the possible future compromise is a floors and ceilings model we have argued for throughout this book using Medicare+Choice for all or the Federal Employees Health Benefits Program model as an alternative.

Health Care Strategies: An Update

Health plans raised rates consistently through 2000 and beyond and began to dig themselves out of the deep financial hole of the mid-1990s. But they are all playing a game of catch-up with a health care delivery system that is flexing its clout and growing again at double-digit rates. The core strategies remain.

- *Vertically integrated for value.* Kaiser is flourishing, in its strong core markets of the West and Hawaii, as a plan that vertically integrates to deliver value to its employer customers and its plan members. Kaiser has returned to its roots of having a unique partnership with the Permanente Medical groups and has bet the farm on redesigning health care delivery using the Internet and sophisticated IT to unite its consumer portal, electronic medical record system, and clinical knowledge base. It remains a formidable competitor in its home markets and will do well in the long run. But it is the Greek Orthodox Church—a different type of medicine. Kaiser has loyal members, physicians, and employees who are true believers. But like Greek Orthodoxy it is not for everyone. The good news for Kaiser is that California is Greece. Attempts to build a more secular Kaiser through the delegated medical group model, advocated by PacifiCare and HealthNet in particular, are perilously close to collapse. This is sad because the large medical group, whether Kaiser Permanente or secular in flavor, is the best hope we have for a source of innovation in how medicine can and should be practiced in the twenty-first century.

- *Virtual single payer.* The virtual single payer model described in Chapter Nine has served the health plans well. The major players who pursued this nationally, including Aetna, CIGNA, and United have done reasonably well. But by far the best examples remain strong regional plans, such as Wellpoint, Highmark, and Anthem, that use their local clout to extract deep discounts and control the game. This model has come under political assault as "the hamster care model" for placing doctors in a virtual discounted fee-for-service hamster wheel: it alienated doctors and patients alike. In turn, this has led all of these plans to renounce utilization management, pursuing instead the new mantra "you can go anywhere and have anything done, but you just might just have to pay more for it." Many of these plans are well positioned, Wellpoint in particular, to build new generations of consumer-tiered products on their existing employer client base and information systems. The Achilles heel for these plans is that their sheer firepower has led to the formation of countervailing power at the hospital level, as we will discuss below.

- *New paradigms.* Self-directed health plans must be the wave of the future because we are attending conferences about them. Actually, that is a pretty good indicator that they will *not* grab the market: witness disease state management and e-health. While many of the new kids on the block (or rather old kids with new companies) have some very interesting ideas, much work and marketing needs to be done to make them a real force. We should welcome the innovation they may spur in the traditional health plan business (a sleepy and tired industry), but we should not expect them to be the key to the future. Rather their ideas will be co-opted and marketed by the virtual single payers who have clout and customers.

- *Value added partner.* The future of the health plan is to transform itself into a value-added partner with its employer customers. In the crudest possible terms, that means that the health plans will help the employers develop sophisticated new ways to screw the employees and get them to pay more of the bill for health care. It will all be coated in kinder, gentler, self-directed, empowerment, market-based gobbledygook, but it will be about the consumer paying more for care. There will be some good things, too. Internet-enabled self-service will actually help the consumer/enrollee navigate through care and insurance choices. New disease management services and medical concierge functions may actually really improve the care of the chronically ill, if done right. And there could actually be some people who connect their lifestyle choices with their health bill and make some appropriate modifications. Although given that 15 percent of patients account for 85 percent of costs, it's hard to believe those poor souls brought it all on themselves. Some of it is just bad genes and bad luck.

Provider Strategies

The biggest shift in the last two years has been the increasing clout of providers. As described earlier in Chapter Ten, the growth of horizontal cartels and benevolent monopolists at the hospital level has been a spectacularly successful strategy in getting the upper hand with health plans, even the all-powerful virtual single payers. No health plan can afford to have a major hospital cartel missing from its offering in an era of choice and patient rights. However, these plans will fight back with new wrinkles, such as tiered hospital copayments described earlier, which may start to influence patient choices of hospital, if not the contracted rate of reimbursement for the services provided.

Even physicians have learned to play monopoly and oligopoly. It is tougher for them because they don't *do* group, and they don't *do* business. But they have found ways. All over the country, thirty-mile regional cartels of anesthesiologists, radiologists, and oncologists have proliferated. They are huddling together not for the efficiency, but for the local market power. On a broader scale, doctors through their state medical associations (Texas and California in particular) have taken on the HMOs on anti-trust and even (in the case of California) racketeering charges. Students of irony will ask the question, Exactly who is holding the racket?

Implications for Leaders

The health care system continues its evolution. But these emerging trends have some important new implications for leaders.

Tiering will continue, and the high end will benefit. In the new future described above you won't be hassled if you want to visit a specialist or have your elective surgery at the fanciest hospital in the country. You will just pay more. And that may be fine and dandy for a tiny sliver of rich Americans. I worry about what this means for working people who have to make real choices between taking the right medication or making a rent payment or car payment or feeding their kids.

Shallower coverage for rising health care costs. Any way you cut it, these trends lead to shallower coverage for rising health care costs. The underinsured will grow substantially, and many people who thought they had good health insurance will find themselves underinsured for the first time.

Consumerization and the Internet offer new business opportunities. The Internet is not dead. In fact, it still represents a major source of innovation and efficiency in how health care is administered and delivered. Medical and service excellence can be enabled through e-commerce, and health care leaders need to embrace these tools to reduce costs, improve quality, and increase responsiveness to customers, just as the major industrial giants such as General Electric are doing.

The innovation imperative. The need for innovation has not diminished. The twenty-year clock is ticking, and the reluctant donkey needs to be moved along. Medical technology will accelerate at an ever-escalating rate as the fruits of molecular biology and the new sciences of nanotechnology and genomics produce ever more powerful tools. The challenge for health care finance and delivery is to keep up.

Connection to community. Leaders at all levels need to remember to connect to their community. Local communities can sustain vulnerable but important institutions. Lose support of your community and you are toast.

Vision, values, and leadership. The redesign of health care in the image of the IOM report represents a useful vision for the future. But the reality is that we will see a more tiered, inequitable health care system emerge in the short run. Given the lack of consensus on core health care values and larger worries about national security, it is unlikely we will take on major policy changes in health care until after 2004. In the interim, it will be easy for a confused public to be appeased by flimsy Medicare drug benefit proposals that don't cost much and don't do much; to be seduced by new-sounding free-at-last health plans that have a surprising sting in the pocket book; and to be swayed by a plethora of new direct-to-consumer marketing of new drugs, technology, and care alternatives. To navigate through this uneasy time will take real leadership—leaders who not only inspire us to follow but who tell the truth and take the heat for it.

The Five Pillars of Leadership

Health care is complex. It is full of professions, guilds, unions, and community stakeholders, all of which make leadership more difficult. How do you lead in such an environment? In conclusion and with some humility, I offer five pillars of leadership.

Pillar One: Distinguish Between Managing and Leading

This is by no means an original thought, but it is at the heart of the health care leadership problem. Health care at all levels, from presidential policy to bedside decisions, is over-managed and under-led. What's the difference? You can do no better, in my view, than John Gardner's definition in his 1990 classic, *On Leadership*. To paraphrase Gardner, leaders distinguish themselves from the general run of managers in at least six respects:

1. They think longer term.
2. They understand the relationship between their organization and the wider environment.
3. They reach and influence stakeholders beyond their own organization's boundaries.
4. They put heavy emphasis on the intangibles of vision, values, and motivation, and they understand intuitively the nonrational and unconscious elements in both leading and following.
5. They have the political skill to cope with the conflicting requirements of multiple constituencies.
6. They think in terms of renewal and adaptation to an ever-changing reality, not just sticking to the system.

Pillar Two: Respect Leadership as a Political Process

Leading an organization is more like running a small country than managing a large store. Leadership is inherently political, which frustrates many promising managers who have been promoted because of high marks, good work performance, and self-righteous excellence. In a world of coalition building, compromise, and horse trading, these managers get frustrated, and many fail as leaders.

Pillar Three: Understand the American Leadership Preference

Americans like reluctant leaders with a casual, easygoing style much more than pushy, formal ones. They like Tom Hanks in *Saving Private Ryan* or Jimmy Stewart in *Mr. Smith Goes to Washington*, not Gordon Gekko of "greed is good" fame. This is why George W. cultivated a "gee shucks" Texan style to play down the Andover, Yale, and Harvard in him.

Pillar Four: Honor Moral Leadership.

A lot has been made of values-based leadership in recent years, but even Attila the Hun had values. When people say values-based leadership, they tend to be implying they have the right values, therefore their position should be followed. I prefer to think about the moral base of leadership. Is your position on the side of the angels (consult your own God here)? Is it life affirming? How would it look on the front page of the *New York Times*? Does it feel right in your gut? And most important, what would your mother say?

Pillar Five: Lead the Revolution

Leading the Revolution, strategy guru Gary Hamel's book, is a must-read about the importance of breakthrough innovation in business strategy. This is Hamel in a nutshell, and in his own words:

> I found that most successful companies were following the polestar of some truly noble aspiration. What counted was not so much how they positioned themselves against longstanding rivals, but how creatively they used their core competencies to create entirely new markets.

Health care desperately needs innovation, not just in process and tools, but in business and organizational design. We need leaders who can imagine a better future and take us there.

About the Author

IAN MORRISON is an internationally known author, consultant, and speaker specializing in long-term forecasting and planning, with particular emphasis on health care and societal change. Morrison has written, lectured, and consulted on a wide variety of forecasting, strategy, and health care topics for government, industry, and various nonprofit agencies in North America, Europe, and Asia. He has worked with more than one hundred Fortune 500 companies in health care, information technology, and financial services. Project sponsors also include the Robert Wood Johnson Foundation, the Commonwealth Fund, the Kaiser Family Foundation, and the World Health Organization. He is a frequent commentator on the future for television, radio, and the print media.

Morrison is the author of *The Second Curve: Managing the Velocity of Change* (Ballantine, 1996), which made both the *New York Times* business best-seller lists and the *Business Week* best-seller list. Morrison has coauthored several books and chapters, including *Future Tense: The Business Realities of the Next Ten Years* (Morrow, 1994); *Reforming the System: Containing Health Care Costs in an Era of Universal Coverage* (Faulkner & Gray, 1992); *System in Crisis: The Case for Health Care Reform* (Faulkner & Gray, 1991); *Directing the Clinical Laboratory* (Field & Wood, 1990); and *Looking Ahead at American Health Care* (McGraw-Hill, 1988). He also has coauthored numerous journal articles for such publications as *Encyclopedia Britannica*, *Across the Board*, *The British Medical Journal*, *New England Journal of Medicine*, and *Health Affairs*.

Morrison was president of the Institute for the Future (IFTF) from 1990 to 1996 and was responsible for leading IFTF's growth and success over that period. Prior to becoming president, Morrison led IFTF's part in Health Care Outlook, an ongoing forecasting service for clients in the health care industry, along with joint venture partners from Louis Harris and Associates and the Department of Health Policy and Management at the Harvard School of Public Health.

Before coming to IFTF in 1985, Morrison spent seven years in British Columbia, Canada. During this time he held positions in consulting, teaching, and research. He holds an interdisciplinary Ph.D. in urban studies from the University of British Columbia; an M.A. in geography from the University of Edinburgh, Scotland; and a graduate degree in urban planning from the University of Newcastle-upon-Tyne, England. He is a member of the board of directors of Interim Services, a leading temporary services company; Oceania, a privately held electronic medical record company; and the Health Research and Education Trust, the research and education arm of the American Hospital Association.

Index

A

Academic medicine, and pursuit of fame, 175–178

Access Plus HMO, 83, 154

Access to health care: global, 93; and health status, 55

Accountability: individual, as U.S. health care value, 4; shift toward, 206

Accountability systems: future direction of, 157–162; global interest in, 95

Accreditation: performance measurement versus, 157; requirements for, 158

Adam Smith Beats Karl Marx— Health Care as Financial Services scenario, 223–226

Advocacy groups, consumerization and, 43–44

Aetna U.S. Healthcare, 20, 62, 195

Aggregators, as source of managed care growth, 145–146

Aid for Families with Dependent Children (AFDC) program, 117

Alternative medicine: consumerization and, 44–45; rise of, 11, 128

Altman, S., 148–149

Ambassadors Program, 73

American Association of Retired Persons (AARP), 106

American Hospital Association (AHA), focus of, 24, 57–58

American Medical Association (AMA), leadership challenges for, 25

American Medical International (AMI), 63

Anderson Consulting, 62

Anthem, 19–20

Applied Materials, 206

Archetypes, health insurance, 96–99

Argentina, three-tiered health insurance system in, 101

Arizona, Medicare risk contracting in, 107

Australia: satisfaction with health care in, 93; socialized insurance archetype in, 97, 99; three-tiered health insurance system in, 101

Automated Data Processing (ADP), 145

B

Baptist Health Systems, 185

Belgium, mandatory health insurance archetype in, 98

Bennett, W., 17

Berwick, D., 206

Blendon, R., 80

Blue Shield of California: Access Plus HMO of, 83, 154; consumer focus of, 43, 154–155; future innovation in, 197; market break given to, 152–153; Web site of, 154

289